Myeloma
and me

Ray Grummett

TO David and Jane

Gratefue thanks for all of your help
and encouragement

Ray

© Ray Grummett 2002
Myeloma and me

ISBN   0-9-540341-1-2

Published by International Myeloma Foundation (UK)
9 Gayfield Square
Edinburgh
Scotland
EH1 3NT

Design & production co-ordinated by:
The Better Book Company Ltd
Havant
Hampshire
PO9 2XH

Printed in England.

Cover design by MusicPrint

FOREWORD
(i) Dr Robert Marcus FRCP FRCPath

This book is a testament to the courage of Mr Raymond Grummett and his family after he was diagnosed with multiple myeloma which is a severely debilitating and potentially fatal disease of the blood and bone marrow. The book describes Mr Grummett's treatment and his feelings with a sense of detachment and humour without minimising the trauma which he has suffered.

Unfortunately the only treatment that we have for patients with cancer in general and myeloma in particular is extremely toxic with major side effects to tissues often not affected by the disease itself. This is because the therapy we have is very non-specific and attacks normal as well as the cancerous tissue. We rely on the body's own powers of regeneration to allow us to give such powerful therapies. Nevertheless such treatment has made a major impact on many cancers including leukaemia, lymphoma and myeloma, but patients do have to suffer considerable distress and physical discomfort whilst receiving this treatment. We very much hope that in the near future specific therapies which will target the cancer cells and leave normal tissues undamaged will be developed. Until that time (and it will not be far off since some antibody therapies are now entering general use) we have to expect that our patients will suffer the rigours of intensive therapy for the sake of long term benefits.

Mr Grummett has written a detailed account which may have helped him to reconcile himself to the unpleasant therapy he has undergone but I hope this book will serve a wider purpose which is to inform patients that, despite the unpleasantness of treatment and widespread side effects, the achievable goal is to attack the cancer and restore the patient to normal health.

I hope other patients with myeloma will read this book and take inspiration from Mr Grummett's courage.

(ii) Dr R. Weare MRCP, MB Chb, MA

This is the diary of one man's experience of the effects and treatment of Multiple Myeloma, a disease currently without a cure.

However, it is more than that.

It describes with clarity, honesty and humour the thoughts and feelings of a man undertaking a journey which was horrific and yet therapeutic. Throughout this experience, he faces bravely the larger issues of life, and finds not only himself, but the true value of others.

This book will be of great value to anyone about to face a similar battle in the future, but I think its value is much wider. Although it is a personal journal, it addresses the qualities and frailties encompassed by being a human.

CONTENTS

ACKNOWLEDGEMENTS

I would like to dedicate this book to the many scientists who are trying to find a cure for this illness. To the medical and nursing teams at Addenbrooke's, The Evelyn, and my Surgery, in fact everyone who looked after me in so many different ways, in particular Doctors Marcus and Weare. To my family and friends who shared this ghastly time with me, but mostly, profoundly, to my wife June without whom this book, and very little else would have been possible.

Disclaimer

Chapter One – The Early Days

Nov. 15th 1994 I have myeloma, cancer of the plasma cells. I have just been told.

Apart from sporting injuries, and minor illnesses such as Chicken Pox, until recently I have had very little to do with doctors, that is clearly going to change, and will take some adjusting to. Although this particular cancer is rare, it is treatable, but at one stroke, we are talking about a serious illness by any definition, a true grown-ups illness. Phrases like life threatening, life shortening, damage to the quality of life, aspirations, biopsies, already, I have decided that Chicken Pox was better.

Any sensible person will have wondered how they would react in these circumstances. I had hoped, particularly when the children were small that if it happened I would at least not let anyone down. It would make the whole thing so much worse if I was terrified and showed it, but logically this was unlikely. All of the male members of my family carry phlegmatism almost to an art form, and I was not expecting much trouble on that score. In the event, numbness took over to an extent, and it made the stiff upper lip easier to effect. When the diagnosis came I was expecting it to be worse, and in a sense, it was a relief.

I can not envisage a situation where a patient (see how quickly the terminology is used) is told of cancer without any warning. If nothing else everyone who has cancer must feel that it is a different illness to anything they have had before. No matter how dim, the patient who undergoes the battery of tests, bone marrow aspirations, biopsies, etc. must have some inkling that all is not well. Step by step the knowledge, doubts, and fears build up until the final diagnosis, which I maintain is not a great surprise when it happens.

What did surprise me, was my initial reaction. It was far too soon to feel the classical "Why me?", "What have I done to deserve this?", etc. I have no religious hang ups and the other classical reaction "God has decreed this never entered my head. If God does visit cancer on family men he must have a warped sense of humour. On the other hand it may be that having a religion can give some strength, but if this is the case I missed out. On the way back from Cambridge in the car, my wife, June must have thought I was being my usual monosyllabic self, but I was thinking about Suman Singh, strange how the mind plays tricks.

Suman Singh was with me in the Royal Air Force during the days of National Service and was memorable for two things. One was his marching ability, and the other was his skill at fortune telling, and reading palms. There are two marching techniques, the standard, and the "farmers boy" where the right arm is thrust forward with the right leg. The theory is that it is caused by walking too much with hands in moleskin trouser pockets, but Suman did a variation of this.

His basic stride was the "farmers boy", but in his case the arm followed the leg slightly more slowly. After 12 strides or so, he was marching properly for a split second, and then the cycle would repeat itself. The Drill Instructors used to bring their colleagues to watch, and they would leave with a wondrous look in their eyes as if they had witnessed a sight seen by very few people, as indeed they had.

The fortune telling and palm reading was what made me remember this as it had a relevance to my illness. Of all the charlatans, crack-pots, cheats, con men, and preyers on simple minds, I would place these people pretty high on the list. I would have nothing to do with the sessions run by Suman, and was amazed at the sheer gullibility of ostensibly rational people.

Each flight intake consisted of 360 fit single young men, interested in young women, sport, enjoyment, and drink, not necessarily in that order. The predictions made by Suman were invariably centred around vague hints of career moves, future friendships with women, and travel. How remarkable, what a gift the man had. I had nothing to do with it, despite raucous encouragement from my friends, until one night I must have had more to drink than usual, and succumbed. He looked at my palm, and blanched, or as near as was possible, and flung my hand down as if it were hot. He backed away, murmuring "Trouble, Trouble" and clearly did not want to take part in the charade any more. I had had a rough upbringing up to that point, and suggested that to him, but he said that it was the future he feared, but would give no further details. Could it be that he had actually seen something, or was he simply getting his own back for the ribald comments he had suffered from me.

So there you are Suman, wherever you are now. You made me remember that incident after all this time, if you feel that you have got your own back for the things I said about you, good luck to you. It changes nothing, I still feel exactly the same about such people and I am not about to let 35 year old mumbo jumbo and clap-trap upset me now.

The myeloma has made me focus more on the effect it could have long term, which is completely new to me. Up to now my health has been excellent, and I had assumed that it would carry on forever. It has always been my aim to live until 100, or die in the attempt. The few illnesses I have had, I knew for certain that within a very short time, I would be cured. This one is clearly different, and it is forcing me to look back at half forgotten things over the last few months.

I developed catarrh, not particularly badly, but bad enough after a few months to consult my G.P. After a few tries, I had largely given up, perhaps conscious of going to see a doctor with something so trivial. This was purely my thoughts, none of the doctors had even hinted this, quite rightly. Anyone who attends the doctor as rarely as I, must by definition be treated seriously when they do go. My own doctor, who I have a lot of time for, said that it may be something that I would have to live with, and that he himself had the same problem. I mentioned that his cigarette smoking may have something to do with it, which he accepted with good grace. Even so we were still no nearer to curing my problem.

Also around this time, I noticed that I was becoming tired more easily. I noticed that people were passing me on pavements, something which had very rarely happened before. I have always been a fast walker, the first thing June does is get hold of my arm, or I am out of sight in no time. Any number of people were quick to say that as I was 55, slowing down was natural, but this was an anathema to me. Every age I have been so far, I have considered myself to be 5 years short of my prime, and it is still so, let others talk themselves into a zimmer frame, not I.

We went to Australia over Christmas 1993, fortified with all the inoculations our surgery could provide, but I developed the worst cold I could remember. I could have done without it as we were meeting our son in law for the first time. As it turned out, it did not matter, as Steve is one of those people who seem to be able to get on well with anyone, spluttering and sneezing notwithstanding. It was great to see my daughter Andie and Steve so obviously happy and settled down, but the cold was cramping my style. Every symptom of a cold I had ever had or heard about was there, not pleasant at all. It was by far the worst cold I had ever had, my white cells must have been on double time.

What made me stop and think at the time, was the afternoon Andie and I went to the viewing platform on Sydney Harbour Bridge. A few years ago although Andie smoked then, I used to beat her at Squash, and here was I, desperately trying to keep up with her climbing the stairs. I managed not to stop, masculine and parental pride being what it is, but it was a close thing. I should have realised then, that I was unfit at the very least.

Shortly after coming home, I noticed that my feet were aching around the ball of my foot, and along the side towards the heel. We went for a short break in the spring and after returning from Ibiza my feet were worse. I put this down to wearing flip-flops, but soon even allowing for my natural reluctance to visit doctors, I found that they had deteriorated to the extent that I had to go. Also, I noticed that small cuts or scratches were taking a long time to heal, in one case many months. Even allowing for the fact that metabolism slows down, this seems to have happened suddenly, dating back from when the catarrh started.

Nothing seemed to help, and at one point, I found that in one of my nocturnal trips, I could not walk diagonally across the bedroom. I had to lean against the wall, and shuffle to the corner, turn along the other wall and reach the door that way. If June had seen me heaven knows what she would have thought, but secret use of alcohol would have been a front runner. I even talked to an Osteopath, and a Chiropodist, but their joint view was a possibility of Morton's Metatarsalgia but to carry on with the present investigations.

I was by then having a series of blood tests, and coincidentally had donated a pint of blood just before. Knowing what was to come, I just hope that the National Blood Transfusion Service do a thorough job on screening blood before it is passed on. After completing the blood tests, my G.P. admitted that he was baffled, and was making arrangements to have me referred. I applaud this, as professional pride must make it a great temptation to try everything before calling in a specialist. Thankfully my doctor referred me quickly, and saved me from deteriorating.

The sting in the tail was that he warned me that it was classed as non-urgent and that the appointment with the specialist may be "some months" away. When I was with the bank, they paid for their managers to join a private health scheme. This was a way of ensuring that managers were away from their desks as little as possible, but it turned out to be a boon to me. I chose to carry this on when I retired, what a good decision to make. I must admit to misgivings over private medicine, with my upbringing I suppose it is hardly surprising. Most of the males in my family were Communists. The remainder were to the left of them. I justified joining by thinking of how I would react if one the children were ill, I just could not bear them having to wait if I had the means to have them treated sooner. For 12 years I have had no need to use the scheme, but it certainly came into its own with this illness.

This is how I came to attend an appointment with the Consultant Rheumatologist, at Rivers Hospital on Sept 27th 1994. She suspected Rheumatoid Arthritis, certainly my feet were getting worse, my maximum range was from home to the Library and back, a total of one mile if that. The pain was such that I was walking badly, which was making my back ache, and the lack of exercise was making me put on weight, and generally, I felt that I was going downhill. Even allowing for my reluctance to put myself in medical hands (this seems crazy being married to a nurse), clearly something had to be done.

The consultant was very thorough, and ordered the full battery of blood tests, X Rays etc. , and as she could see no reason to cancel, we went to Northern Majorca that weekend for an autumn break. The idea was that the results of the various tests would be completed by the time we returned. At this point farce took over.

On the day we were to go, I developed a massive nose bleed which took over 2 hours to stop. It happened again at work, and again when I got home. Then in the evening, June started with diarrhoea and sickness, and when the time came to go to the airport, it was touch and go. Paul, (No 2 son) gave us a lift, and on stepping out of the car, my nose started again. An impressive sight we were waiting to check in. June scurrying off every few minutes, me with tissue rammed up the nose to stem the flow of blood, and kicking the cases along in the general direction of the check in desk. The other passengers were quite amused, and no doubt had christened me "the bleeder", June's description is best left to the imagination. Strange how nose bleeds had never bothered me in the past, but in the near future, problems with blood was to dominate my life.

The holiday was to be relaxing, and in terms of what I was able to do, it could not have been anything else. I tried to swim, but it was as if someone was hammering at my little toes with a cold chisel. Nothing I could do was any help, I can do three swimming strokes equally badly, and the pain was the same in all three, so no swimming. Walking was getting to be a torment, my level of exercise was reducing, the level of fitness was reducing, and the only thing increasing was my girth. I could always eat, and the weight was piling on. I had visions of going home like a Toby jug.

All of this I was blaming on the state of my feet, even the exhaustion, which I was attributing to the lack of general fitness. Having almost never been ill, I had no experience to draw on, but in retrospect, one black day should have made me think a little harder. We decided to visit the next bay which was about 3 miles, in normal times, we would walked without giving it a second thought. On this day the walk to the bus stop was about a quarter of a mile, and I was played out when I got there. The Spanish drivers had elected to go on siesta, and this of course took precedence over the timetable.

We stood for over an hour, and I could do little else when we arrived than go for a coffee. No buses back, no sign of taxis and yet another interminable wait until the drivers decided that they had had enough sleep. It made it worse when it became obvious that our Courier had known of this siesta and had not told us. It confirmed my view of him when he told me a story concerning football results. I always try to find out the Sunderland result wherever I am and he told me that he copied the scores down from the radio. One day he ended up with one team short, so he simply missed it out and put the sheet up on the notice board. I can imagine the absolute chaos that would have caused.

The point of all this is that my level of tiredness was certainly exhaustion, and I should have been suspecting that things were not good. Dragging myself back to our room was getting to be the norm, and yet after a short rest, I could cope again very well. There remains however, a dividing line between being tired, and being exhausted and on many occasions I was crossing this line, and looking back should have been aware of it. I did realise that whatever was bothering me was something I had never had before, but still put it down to my feet.

This mistaken impression lasted only for a few days longer. On returning home on October 8th, a letter was waiting, I was to see the consultant again on the 11th. This appointment was short, she told me that she had been beavering away during the week of my holiday, and although the x-rays were clear, an abnormality in the blood had showed up on the tests. This took it out of her speciality, and she had discussed it with the Haematologist at Harlow who thought it best if I go to Dr Marcus at the Evelyn Hospital at Cambridge. I thought it strange that one specialist should refer to another in the same branch of medicine. Apparently Dr Marcus specialises in what they think my problem might be, and that he was the right person to go to. It is all very well to have the best man available, but why is it necessary? In the opinion of my Consultant, Dr Marcus would want to have a look at my bone marrow. I was to learn very quickly how nicely doctors and hospitals describe procedures, if euphemisms are a subject in the medical examinations, I would expect a number of 100% pass marks.

I said that I was concerned as an uncle had died of Leukaemia, and she became a little ill at ease. Perhaps in her own field she was not faced with life threatening diseases, but it seemed that my remark had shaken her composure for a moment. She offered to fax the results that day if I could fix up an appointment, in the event, I was able to see Dr Marcus on October 13th and called for the letter that day. Certainly, speed was of the essence, and I was aware of this, but was not sure if this was the difference between the N.H.S. and private medicine.

Apart from a football injury which turned out to be the same as Brian Clough's and years later Paul Gascoine's, my experience of hospitals had been nil. Nevertheless, here was I, an ex Chicken Pox sufferer, being sent off to Cambridge in what seemed to me in an almost indecent haste. Things were getting out of my control. I had a fleeting thought that it was my G. P. getting his own back, teaching me a lesson for bothering him with my bad feet. "I'll give the bugger something to think about". It certainly stopped me worrying about my feet for a while.

13 October 1994

The Evelyn Hospital seemed to me to be impressive, albeit with my less than vast experience, a lovely old building modernised with taste. Dr Marcus it turns out is a Consultant Haematologist at the Addenbrooke's, so far so good. He is younger than I had expected, quietly spoken, with no trace of obsequiousness, a professional who answered our questions as well as he was able. Clearly he was not going to make guesses at this early stage, and would need to know some facts before doing so. This step by step approach is without doubt correct, but the average impatient patient has to learn to accept this very early.

After an early chat and the noting of my medical history the process seemed to move forward of its own volition. Dr Marcus said that my original blood tests showed a few cells that he would need to find out more about. He said that he would need to carry out more tests, and would like a look at my bone marrow. When I asked him when he said "Well, now", and seemingly without any action on my part I was lying on an examination table trying my level best not to look at any needles or equipment. I have managed over the years to donate blood regularly, and never once in 36 years have I looked at what they were doing.

Whether it is normal practice, or if they picked up my nervousness I am still unsure, but the procedure was preferable to visiting a dentist, certainly a dental hygienist. There was no pain, but a discomfort throughout. This was made much better by both Dr Marcus and his nurse telling me what was going on, it is so much better than being left in the dark. I was told when an uncomfortable point was reached, and how long it would take, and I found this to be so helpful.

Hearing about procedures such as Lumbar Punctures in the past, I had doubted if I could actually submit to it, but after 20 minutes or so, I had completed my ordeal, and had endured as close to the dreaded L. P. as I would wish. More discussion with Dr Marcus before leaving for x-rays, but already I am picking up his style. Absolutely no flannel, he said that he would see the results of the bone marrow test, and left me in no doubt that he would get to the bottom of it, and decide the best course of treatment. Again, I have no way of knowing, but in my case, even before diagnosis, we are linking illness with treatment, and I found this reassuring.

The slight unease returned in the x-ray department, as it became clear to me that the department had been kept behind for me. This started the brain cells working again, asking why was the whole thing being done in such a rush. The appointment, the bone marrow extract and now the x-ray were clearly designed to have the results back in the shortest time possible. No doubt this is the ideal situation for all patients, but it did leave a lingering doubt in my mind. Was this the difference between private medicine and the N.H.S., or was there some hidden agenda. With my knowledge of medical procedures I had no way of knowing.

The drive home was subdued, I have never regarded myself as being stupid, and I knew that bone marrow samples are not taken lightly. June, on the other hand would be way ahead of me, already thinking of the possibilities, and neither of us wanting to put it into words. I was very much aware that the boys would be home, and I would have to take a decision as to what to tell them. Ian and Paul had made sure that they would be there when we got home, and would expect some information. Again with my family being so healthy previously, they had no idea what to expect and would be anxious.

In common with most parents, I find it difficult to regard my own children as anything else but kids, and this is nonsense. Paul is the youngest at 21, the three of them are adults, fine young people, of whom we can be justifiably proud. It would be insulting to hide anything from them, but at this time we know nothing, suspected a little more, and feared a little more still. All I could tell them was that the tests were proceeding, and that we would know in a few days time what had been found. I had no problem with this approach, as the lads could see that I was well on the face of it, but Andie was another problem. With her living in Australia, I could see little benefit in telling her that I could be seriously ill, far better to wait until I knew what, if anything was wrong, and tell her then.

1 November 1994

Back to the Evelyn, another lovely day. At least if I had the worry of another consultation, we had a pleasant drive to make up for it. Dr Marcus welcomed June to sit in again, which suits me fine. She can understand the medical terms, and I find it far better that two of us are there to minimise the risk of anything being forgotten. It may be just me, but I find that my brain goes into atrophy, and if all patients are similar, it must be very hard for consultants not to assume that the population at large have an I.Q. of 10.

There is still no firm news, which is at once a relief, and disappointing. On the basis that it is far better to travel hopefully than to arrive, there is a sense of relief, but we have resolved nothing. Dr Marcus is still not certain, but is able to tell us that there are rogue cells in the marrow, but he is not sure how active they are, and therefore can not be sure what treatment is required if at all. Again, the linking of treatment and diagnosis is reassuring, plus the knowledge that whatever it is, can not be rampaging round my blood, or it would be more apparent. To take us a step further, he has arranged that I attend the Nuclear Medicine Department at Addenbrooke's for a liver function test.

I have started to wake up during the night, around four in the morning is the worst time. This is apparently the time when most people die, and I can see why. Any slight problem is magnified a hundred times, and the worry about my future diagnosis was looming large. Strangely, I had never thought about dying from this illness, whatever it was but the horrors seemed to be all financial. I had black moments about not being able to work any more, and being dependant on my pension to get Paul through University. I convinced myself at one stage that we would have to sell the house and move downmarket away from our friends, never have holidays any more, give up the car, all sorts of nonsense. If I was unable to get back to sleep, I would read, the girls at the library must have thought I was on a speed reading course. If I could not get back to sleep, then, I was grateful for the birds singing to take my mind off things. Four in the morning is when people are at their lowest ebb, I can vouch for that.

11 November 1994

The liver function test involves placing a Radio-Isotope in a vein, and plotting the flow through the liver, by way of repeated blood tests. A thought did occur that a cheaper, and more pleasant way would have been to use a few pints of Abbot. This could be because they have not yet been told that P.P.P. are paying, the needles and blood job could be N.H.S.

The actual procedure turned out to be boring. A separate puncture had to be made for each blood collection, but this was no worse than blood doning, and I had voluntarily endured that since I was 19. The radioactive material was inserted by an Australian doctor, so at least we had something to talk about to divert me from what he was doing. I then had to return in 2 hours time for another blood sample, then again in 1 hour, and finally in another hour. Hence the boredom. My tame Australian did say that the test was to determine how much chemotherapy I would need. This was the first mention of specific treatment, although I would need to have been brain dead not to have seen the possibility. Various options were open. Either he knew something we did not, or he simply assumed that the treatment would be required, or Dr Marcus had found the diagnosis since we saw him. Either way, events seemed to be moving of their own free will. This left me still feeling perfectly well, with potentially a serious illness, and feeling like the mythical Manuel, knowing nothing. I say feeling perfectly well, this is of course, apart from my wretched feet, which is how the whole thing started.

I have been stumbling around rather than walking properly for some months. I have been walking stooped, and this is making me unfit, as I can not exercise properly. The walk to collect my paper is getting to be the limit of what I can do. Old ladies are passing me with shopping trolleys going up hill, I am now dreading having to walk anywhere instead of looking forward to it. The low point up to now was having to make a nocturnal visit some nights ago. I found the pain so bad that I could not go diagonally across the room but had to support myself against the walls to reach the door. This was causing me far more worry than the tests I was undergoing as nothing seemed to be logical. There seemed to be no difference if I rested or tried to operate normally, it made no difference what shoes I wore, but it was always worse in the mornings and after standing for long periods.

I was still carrying on working, but found that I had to lecture sitting down rather than at a lectern, which to be honest made little difference. The Bench also posed few problems although the Lord Chancellor decided to get into the act. 1994 was the first year that new Chairmen had to be trained and assessed, and all of this had to be completed by the end of November. This meant that on the days when I was to be assessed, I had to be there, and it meant juggling hospital visits with days when my feet were particularly bad. At least it focused a problem which we needed to sort out.

When Magistrates leave court, it has never been resolved in what order they should leave. Should it be Chairman first, ladies first, the one nearest the door first, or in my case the one with the worst limp goes last? The consensus is now that the person nearest the door goes first, but chivalry dies hard. I remembered from years ago a suggested method of contraception, which was to put a stone in your shoe, and that would make you limp. I must remember to ask Dr Marcus if a rapidly deteriorating brain is a possible symptom.

In the context of trying to alleviate the boredom of filling in the time between blood tests, we took to walking around the hospital. The Nuclear Medicine Department is near to the Outpatients Department, but this is at the opposite end of the hospital to the concourse where the main cafeteria is situated. We walked to the main concourse for lunch, and found that it was taking 15 minutes, and whilst Addenbrooke's is a big hospital, it should have taken less than five minutes. The walking was getting me down. A further disappointment was later in the day at home. On my trips to the toilet, at the very least I had expected a Willy that glows in the dark after all the radioactive liquid, but no such luck. Altogether a boring and fruitless day, but at least a further step nearer to finding out what is wrong with me, apart from the damned feet, which inevitably will have to take a back seat to the major problem, as yet unknown.

Chapter Two – Enter The Chemo Kid

15 November 1994

I return to D-Day, Diagnosis day. Again, never having been in this situation before, I had no idea what to expect. Certainly no histrionics, or dramatic phrases on the lines of "I am afraid I have to tell you", or "I have some bad news for you". All the way through Dr Marcus has said that when he knew the facts, he would tell us, and that is what he did. It may that he always uses this technique, or it may be that he had decided it was best for us, but whichever, it was the correct approach. Straight from the shoulder, calm and professional. Up to this point, I had been toying with the daft idea that I could be suffering from a typing error. For "There is evidence of myeloma", read "There is no evidence of myeloma". No such luck.

To say that I felt pleasure in finding out is clearly ridiculous, but it seemed to be more than relief. Relief certainly in finding out what it was, although to confess, it was the first time I had heard the word myeloma used. Relief also, as I had been thinking it was Leukaemia, and as I found out later, June had been thinking at the very beginning, more on the lines of Cancer of the bones. Both of us therefore were able to follow the clinical explanations in a positive, if not relaxed frame of mind.

Myeloma if left unchecked, produces an excess of abnormal proteins, and creates craters in the bones. This makes sense of the full Skeletal x-rays and liver function tests. In the later stages it causes pain and incapacity, luckily mine was in the early stages and no damage could be detected. The illness can lie dormant for years and suddenly become active. Dr Marcus could not be sure if mine was still at the dormant stage, but suspected that it was starting to move. The options were to leave it alone for a while, to contain it by drugs, or to try and eradicate it.

Apparently, it could be contained for many years at the present stage, but having already talked it over with June, we had decided that whatever it was, we wanted rid of it. I was able therefore at a very early stage to indicate my feelings. The choice was really mine and whatever option I had decided Dr Marcus would have gone along with. When I told him my opinion, using my half baked knowledge of body language, I was sure I had chosen correctly, and that was the answer he wanted. The treatment was for a cocktail of drugs, combined with courses of chemotherapy over four months, and assuming I had no bad reactions, to enter hospital for an intensive treatment of chemo, which would hopefully get rid of it once and for all. So it was that right from the start, I had locked horns with this myeloma. Dr Marcus' approach had always been to link diagnosis with treatment, even before the word cancer had settled in, it was on its way out.

The drive home was a bit morose even so, I was a little numb, June was concentrating on driving, and I had my flashback to Suman Singh to rationalise. It may have been the body's response to the unpleasant present to revert to years ago, similar to a faint in similar circumstances. We made a decision not to hide my illness from anyone. Cancer is nothing to be ashamed of. The boys can see that ostensibly I am well, and both have inherited my phlegmatism, but Andie still was a problem. If it would have saved her, and the rest of the family grief, I would quite happily have lied in my back teeth, but it simply was not necessary. If the situation had been that I had, say 12 months to live, then there would have been no point telling her now and letting her worry unduly. We had the information from the hospital to read over and digest, and we could then tell Andie and Steve after sending photographs over to show how well I was looking. The cancer I have is rare, but treatable, and there are many worse things I could have.

Cancer is a frightening word, but mostly because people of my age remember grandparents and older family members dying from it years ago. The advances made in recent years have been staggering, I was to find out later just how true this was. Also, the particular strain of the disease I have is, from what I can gather, one of the more "user friendly" ones. It is not disfiguring, as skin cancer could be. It does not affect eating, I have no pain, and certainly so far, I feel perfectly fit. The side effects of the treatment may get to me later on, but many of the cancers, even the treatable ones would have caused me a lot more trouble, if I have to have a cancer, I will settle for this one. Other diseases apart from cancer fill me with horror. Motor Neurone Disease, or Alzheimer's would frighten the life out of me, I would not take too well to Parkinson's either. I will settle for what I have, and meet it head on.

As I had known both of the lads were home when we returned, and I suspect that they had realised that my illness was potentially serious, and therefore like June and myself, were at least half prepared. They could see that I was looking well, and once we were able to tell them that it was treatable, and that the success rate was high, they took it very well. Their inherited phlegmatism was helpful, certainly Paul is calm whilst Ian is my clone. That lad is so much like I was at his age it is frightening, I hope he has picked up a few characteristics from his mother to counteract the obvious traits he has picked up from me. We agreed to tell Andie when the time is right, and the dreaded hurdle of telling the children was over without too much anxiety. Relatives and friends would have to come later, but the major hurdle was over.

In trying to gauge people's reactions to my illness, I was taken aback at the depth of feeling. The word 'love' has been taken over by the writers of slushy songs and the 'luvvies' who love everyone and all audiences. I found that a better word is bond. When news of my illness spread, it was as if there was a worldwide net which was tightening around me and my family. There is a bond which is between family and friends, which comes out plainly in times like this. It surprised me, but I welcomed it, and it certainly helped.

June went off to work, leaving me to read over the information given to us by the hospital. As I had never heard the word myeloma before, it was all new to me, but it confirmed my impression that there are many worse cancers than this one, and it is preferable to many other non cancerous illnesses.

In the middle of my reading, June came home from work in tears and had been sent home early as she was close to crumbling and could not cope. This staggered me firstly as she had seemed to be coping very well, but secondly came with the realisation that my illness would have a deep effect on other people. June was being upset by the classic questions and observations, such as, "Why is it me who gets this disease?", "What have I done to deserve it?", "It is so unfair", etc. Possibly her level of knowledge was causing her a problem. If a little knowledge is a dangerous thing, then a lot of knowledge must be harrowing.

Certainly up to this point, I had no such feelings. Having almost no religious leanings, any suggestion of "God's will" had no bearing, and I could not countenance any thoughts that I had done something to deserve it. My firm belief on this illness, as with most other major trials in life is that it is just rotten bad luck. Within that bad luck, however is contained the good luck that my cancer is treatable, and the treatment is already being planned. I have noticed other things in my life so far that I have been unlucky to be involved in, but lucky to get out of. I hope this is the same.

Around this time, I was wondering how the myeloma is picked up. Apparently the cause is unknown, but research is continuing. Perhaps if it had been more of a "fashionable" illness like AIDS more money would be spent. I keep thinking back to the onset of my catarrh, and the awful cold I had in Australia when my white cells must have been working at full stretch. At this time they would have been fully occupied, and could have let the myeloma gain access. This may cause a wry smile to the medics, but if they don't know what causes it, then they don't know what doesn't.

Dr Marcus is to let me know when the first treatment is to take place. He even offered to defer it until after Christmas if I wished, which is good news in itself. If the myeloma cells were getting out of control, he would have been pushing for early treatment. Even so, I could see no advantage in waiting. It could mean that Christmas would be spoiled, but we have no young children, and therefore Christmas is largely irrelevant. My feelings were clear, the treatment will have to take place, even if it may be unpleasant, so let us get on with it. My Geordie genes came to the fore, "let's get stuck into it", the medical staff and my family are united in this. Everyone is on the same side, and I am starting to feel sorry for this myeloma. It has no chance at all.

The treatment will be the infusion of various fluids and the first step is to fit a catheter into a vein which would make it far easier on me in the long run. I therefore reported to Addenbrooke's for a central line to be fitted, and this was the first time I had been to a hospital for treatment, apart from my football injury. Ward C10 is like a magnet, right at the top of the building, drawing me all the way up in the lift, past the Kay Kendall plaque, and trying not to dwell on her experience. She was a very attractive, vivacious girl who was to die from Leukaemia at a ridiculously early age. I had to report to the sister, but there was no sister on duty, I suppose it was a good way to meet a number of other nurses quickly. Over the next few months, I will be having numerous trips to C10 and I found the staff to be unfailingly cheerful and helpful, a great benefit to me.

I had been introduced to euphemisms before, along came another. My doctor turned out to be a lovely girl, very pleasant and reassuring, and she told me that the insertion of the central line would not be painful but could be uncomfortable. This was typical Scottish understatement, and at one time I thought it was London Transport's Central Line going in. I knew of course that it was essential, and by summoning up all of my macho stiff upper lipness, managed to stay still long enough to get the thing in.

The only alternative to the line would have been for a new needle to be used each time, and this would have been impossible for me. I was pleased to find the line popping out of my chest with a bright plastic end on, all ready for the chemo, antibiotics, saline, cups of tea, or whatever. Neatly stitched to my chest after a few minutes it felt like it had been there forever. Although I would consider my performance to have been slightly wimpish, I was so pleased that it was all over, and I was so pleased that they let June come in with me. I half pretended that I wanted her to be able to tell me what it was like afterwards, but it wasn't that at all. I simply wanted her near me, and her presence now and many times in the future was a godsend.

Now it was time for the treatment to begin, and I was pleasantly surprised to receive my "Walkman". This was an infusion pump which can hang on a belt or a strap over the shoulder. It bleeps away merrily, feeding a tiny amount of chemo at a time, and allows the wearer to carry on pretty much a normal life. This was the first time I had been able to get my own back on the myeloma. When the chemo started to flow, I allowed myself the satisfaction of thinking, "take that you swine, see how you like that".

I imagined all the myeloma cells had faces on them of people I didn't like. Saddam Hussein, Yasser Arafat were the first, but I expanded this to television performers. I admit I have never met them, but they deserve to be judged on their acts. All of the game show hosts were in there, Cilla Black, Bruce Forsyth, Michael Barrymore, I just imagine their little myeloma faces contorting when the chemo hit them. Noel Edmonds was in there, how he can earn £4m a year doing what he does is mystifying. It was a strange feeling not knowing if the treatment was doing any good. I had never had any symptoms, so I had nothing to go by.

The cassette is unobtrusive, it was simply a case of remembering to keep my arms on the outside of the tubes. Only once when dressing, did I have my arm inside the tubes, and was lucky I did not tear the line out when I raised my arms. The routine settled down to a visit to Addenbrooke's, for the new pump to be fitted, and then wait for the chemo to empty, usually in a week. Then I had a rest for two weeks, and the process would start again.

The only problem it gave me , was one day I got in from work, and the alarm went off. I had to get back to Addenbrooke's , and although I had set up a contingency plan for drivers, as it was near Christmas, I failed to contact anyone. Eventually June came in, and we once again headed for Addenbrooke's, the car was driving itself up the motorway. The nurses managed to check the batteries, and the pump itself, but the alarm went on. One of the girls noticed that when I bent my arm, the alarm stopped, which could suggest a fault in the central line itself. They re-positioned the line, re-stitched it to my chest, and it worked beautifully, never to give me any more trouble.

I had the cassette under my clothes, and no one noticed a thing getting on and off buses, and in and out of cars provided I had it sited properly, and not round my back where I would sit on it. This was not possible at work, however, as I could not keep a coat on indoors. I had wondered on peoples reactions as I already had been surprised. People, myself included do not know how to confront illness in others. In a few cases, people crossed the road rather than talk to me, clearly they were debating whether to speak or not and took the easy way out. I imply no criticism, as I was no better, hopefully I have a better idea now.

At work, the course participants noticed the cassette, and I heard them whispering about it. There seemed no point to try and keep it a secret, so I made a point at the start of every course, to explain what it was. It then became simply an interesting topic of conversation, and served to break the ice. Whilst I would not recommend all lecturers to use the same method, I would say that my explanation of my illness and my cassette offended no one, and gave the course an identity.

I am sure that if anyone is in a quandary over mentioning an illness, just talk about it in a matter of fact way, and everyone will benefit.

The problem normally is that people have no idea if I am happy to talk about it. They then often take the easy way out and say nothing. It is therefore, in my view the responsibility of the person who is ill to bring the subject up in a normal conversational way. Close friends and family know my ideas on the subject and we have never had any difficulty in visiting each other or telephoning. The problems arise with acquaintances, fellow committee members and the like who may have known me for years, but not very well. It is this group who are in a quandary whether to mention it and risk upsetting me, or pretend they are not aware of it, sadly the odd one has avoided me.

I heard a lovely one-liner at my snooker club. My prowess at the game is somewhat less than that of Steve Davis, but one night I hit a purple patch, putting down the last four colours to win the game. My friends were as amazed as I, and I heard one of them say, "That bugger must be on drugs".

All in all the time with my cassette passed off well. It hardly bothered me at all, and a few people called me 'The chemo Kid'. The possible side effects I was warned to look out for did not materialise. There was a horrible metallic taste in my mouth, and although my appetite was unaffected, my sense of taste was. The steroids caused me to be constipated and to gain weight, and until December 18th, this was the sum total of my problems. This was the day my hair started to fall out, and by Christmas it was all gone. This did not bother me as I knew it would happen, but I was surprised at the speed. I was also surprised at the way it came out I had expected to see the odd coil on my pillow, but instead there were great piles of hair. The inside of my shirt collar was like a rats nest, a truly horrible sight.

Vanity has never been one of my faults, so the changed appearance did not bother me, it was the cold that got to me. I had to fight my corner on the choice of headgear, although I conceded the need. I insisted on a "cheese cutter" in preference to the "breton" styles favoured by the young. The only headgear I possessed at the time was a Sunderland AFC baseball cap, and an Australian bush hat complete with corks, neither of which were deemed to be suitable by the style police.

My friends who had not known of my illness did a "double take" which was quite funny at the time. I was still doing my stint as a Magistrate, and one of the prosecutors was fascinated and could not take her eyes off my head. She probably ended the day with crossed eyes and a headache. The chemo had also caused my face to swell and I looked quite cherubic. My face has always been a little gaunt and now that it was fatter, a few people said that I looked better than I did before. I used to describe my face as cadaverous, funny how I have stopped using that expression now.

It was during a court session that I had my first uneasy sensation. A defendant was due to appear to answer bail, and did not attend. The options were to order an arrest warrant with bail, or without bail. After conferring with my colleagues, I made the announcement, "The court will", and that was as far as I got, my brain seized up. Luckily, the court clerk rescued me, but I was shaken. I now know how comedians and actors feel when it happens to them. The clerk realised that I had dried up in seconds, but to me it felt like half an hour and certainly no one else in court was aware, but it is not a nice feeling.

It happened to be a day when I had to go for a new cassette, and I mentioned it to one of the doctors. He said, "Ray, don't let that bother you, I am 26 years old and I am not ill, and I forget names all the time". It was designed to make me feel better, and it did, but at the same time, I knew that my performance in court was poor and that it must be the effect of the treatment. There would shortly come a time when I would have to give up the Bench, work, my committee work, and my role as a School Governor but I was determined to put off the day as long as I could. From that time I started to take more notice of what was happening to me.

There was a regular source of information from Dr. Marcus and his team, as I had reached a critical stage. I had by now had three chemo treatments by way of my cassette, and it was time for the results to be evaluated. I needed to show that I was tolerating the chemo, and that I was getting a good reaction to it, otherwise there would be no point going to Addenbrooke's for the intensive stage. Luckily June could decipher it, but the white cell count was dropping steadily as the chemo wreaked its havoc. I was becoming more and more tired, and although it was easy to sit down and lecture, I felt that I was losing my edge. My memory was certainly not as good, I had more memory lapses on minor things like forgetting footballers names, and it added up to a sense of losing control.

Right from the start, I had resolved to tackle this thing head on, make no concessions to it, and give it no quarter. I knew that once the white count reached a certain level, that I would have very little resistance to disease, and that I would need to stop work, and my other activities. To continue to come into contact with other people with the usual winter colds when I had an immune system that was performing less and less would be lunacy.

At this time we heard from Dr Marcus, and he tells us that apparently, things are going well. This means that we will stop at the 4th chemo, and there will be no need to have any more before being admitted to Addenbrooke's. This will be for the intensive treatment, followed by a Stem Cell Transplant, which was completely new to me. A stem cell is a young blood cell before it matures and becomes a red cell, a white cell, or a platelet. The procedure will be to remove some of my stem cells, purify them, destroy the malignant cells in the bone marrow, and then transplant my own cells back. Written down like this, it seems so straightforward, I hope it turns out that way. The positive side is that I have been tested, and found to be suitable for the next stage which must be good.

By the middle of March, my performance was declining, and although none of my colleagues said they recognised it, I knew the time had come. I stopped work almost at the time the hospital said that I must, the timing was excellent. I stopped taking Courts, which was hard as they are always short of men, and Chairmen. Just before I stopped taking courts, I had to send a defendant to prison. I say had to, as all the Magistrates I know only send people to prison as a very last resort, but in this case I had no option. As he turned to go, he said 'I hope you get cancer and die'. The whole Court hushed, and looked at me. All I could do was shrug my shoulders and carry on, his best line in invective was wasted. Also, my role as School Governor had reached a critical point. In my capacity as Chairman of the Estates committee, I had to consider the provision of new buildings, and I knew that my white cell count was getting very low. I made sure that we took a formal decision to go ahead with three projects that we had been trying to get off the ground for years. This meeting proved to be the last for almost a year, but more of that later. By withdrawing from my activities, it felt in a strange way that I was giving up, but the decision was perfectly sensible.

The chemo up to this point had been designed to weaken the myeloma, and had not given me a great deal of trouble, in fact it had a beneficial effect in cutting down the shaving. I suppose that up until this time I was doing so well I was becoming a little cocky. My outlook was certainly more than positive or optimistic. I thought at the time of the marketing possibilities if the chemo could be controlled and refined. I even thought of an advertising slogan. Just think – "Men do you want to stop shaving for life, eradicate nasal hair for all time, take chemo for Men in handy sachets", "Ladies, banish superfluous hair, and finish with leg shaving and bikini lines – take Chemo Femme". "If you object to your man's hairy back, slip some Chemo for Men in his food", the possibilities are endless.

I was now waiting to go into Addenbrooke's for stage 2 of the treatment, and was feeling confident and impatient to get it over with. My weight was ballooning with the steroids and I will detest steroids for as long as I live. Taking 26 pills a day was an ordeal for someone not used to it, but how people take any kind of drugs voluntarily simply defeats me. Drug taking for so called pleasure must be one of the most stupid things that it is possible to do. I heard a good expression in Court recently about drug taking: "It is not bad because it is illegal, it is illegal because it is bad". As my weight increased, so my energy decreased, I was feeling the effect of the drugs I was taking and becoming more impatient by the day.

I had to go to Addenbrooke's for the function tests before admission. That was lung, liver, kidney, and x-rays and a very useful chat to Gilda Bass, the Transplant Co-ordinator. She was excellent and talked through the possible side effects of the chemo, which in my state of hyper optimism I did not believe applied to me. She also explained that the transplant procedure required a double line and without knowing who suggested it, we agreed to have that done immediately to save time. It was part of Gilda's role to allay fears, instil confidence, and cheer people up. I was so cocky and confident that it turned out to be an enjoyable chat, but with valuable information thrown in. She touched on finances very briefly as that was not one of my problems, but I shuddered to think how I would feel if it was. Just imagine if a patient was worried about the cancer, the treatment and had money worries as well, it doesn't bear thinking about.

It seemed sensible to go on to the ward, have the central line removed, and then a Quinton line would be "slipped in". The "uncomfortable" procedure became quite an ordeal, but one which had to be endured. The local anaesthetic either wore off, or was not up to the job, but it was a grim 20 minutes. I felt sorry for the young doctor. It seemed that it fell to her to do the unpleasant things to me. Having a chivalrous nature and the fact that she looked so young made me sorry for her. She helped by telling me a story of her time in Glasgow in casualty. A huge Scot came in needing stitches after a bottle fight, and insisted on an experienced doctor to look after him. It was Isobel's first night and first stitching job, what a good job her patient never found out. When my new line was safely in, I could appreciate the sense of having it done now, I just wish I could stand the pain a bit better. Wimps of the world unite.

March 1995

Phase 2 is about to begin. At least I am going into hospital for the first time with the right attitude, at least in my opinion. Confidence bordering on cockiness with an aggressive attitude towards the myeloma- have Quinton line will travel.

I arrived at the hospital on the 4th March which happened to be a Saturday, feeling more concerned about the Sunderland game that day than the treatment. Even when I was told that this chemo was very much more powerful that the first stage, I was not particularly concerned. After all the first course did not bother me, so why should this. What a boon ignorance is.

The plan now is for more chemo to kill the myeloma cells in my bone marrow. Stem cells will be collected from my blood, cultured and then stored. The cells will be eventually transplanted back into the bone marrow with no myeloma cells and that should be that. It sounded quite simple, but the reality was more involved, and depended on a fair degree of co-operation all round.

After the two days of stronger chemo, I was allowed to go home. The reason for this was the fact that peripheral blood cells are present in the bone marrow but tend to stay there. Very few find their way into the blood. By regular injections of GCSF, this will dramatically increase the numbers of stem cells, and force them into the blood, from whence they can be collected.

Each day, I had to have injections into my stomach, and luckily I had June available to do it. I am sure that I could never had given them to myself, I have a great admiration for Diabetes sufferers, I couldn't do it. The best part of having your wife to do injections is the absence of any macho pretence. Injections can be done quickly or slowly, and my theory was the quicker the better, and get it over with. The boy's a fool. After the first one, which had me crawling on the ceiling, June did them very slowly, which I found suited me, and I felt no compelling reason to act brave. The blood sample was taken straight to the Path. Lab. at the nearest Hospital, Princess Alexandra's at Harlow, to be analysed, and the results faxed to Ward C10 at Addenbrooke's.

I had to be available to go in at very short notice, as when the white cell count reached the required level, treatment had to start very quickly. When the cells were forcing their way out of the bone marrow, I was warned that it would be a little uncomfortable. This was before I learned the true meaning of the word euphemism, and I was surprised how painful it was. Wimps of the world unite.

Very shortly after this, the prescribed level was reached, we got a phone call from the hospital just before lunch, and we were there by early afternoon. The next stage, had I been an engineer, would have made common sense, but I am not, and I thought it was amazing. My blood was extracted, and rotated in a centrifuge. As each different cell has a different density and weight, it is possible to select exactly what is needed, and replace the remainder. As the various cells were hived off the centrifuge had different colours in bands, I was only sorry I could not see it, This was the reason for the Quinton line which has two ports. One line was taking the cells needed for the transplant, the other was replacing the remaining cells back into my body.

We were left with two bags of peripheral blood stem cells, which would be purified, cultured to provide the transplant team with the required amount, and then deep frozen. The beauty of this procedure is that when the time arrives for the transplant, my own cells would be used and hence no problems with rejection. Not for the first time, I was grateful to the people who had developed this procedure, and the highly competent people who administer it.

My part in this operation was over for the time being, I was sent home once more until the cells were ready for transplantation. Friends and family were calling to see how I was, and were greatly surprised when I answered the phone. The impatience I had previously had abated somewhat. I now knew what was going to happen, and knew that a crucial part of the treatment had already taken place, and I settled down to wait for the next stage, probably in two weeks

4 April 1995

The big day. This time I reported to the ward knowing that this was for the final contest between me and the myeloma. All of the preparations went smoothly, almost as if the medical staff had done it all before. The drugs protocol looked formidable, and there is clearly a balancing act between them. One drug may be essential for anti-sickness, but it would irritate the liver, so another drug was necessary to counteract this, and so it went on. Very important was the need to urinate very often to flush out the kidneys, I had diuretics and fluid through my line and took an amazing amount of fluid on board. I seemed to be trotting off to the toilet every 15 seconds, and had visions of a volunteer force bringing fresh bottles. Not for the first time I was grateful for the provision of a single room for everyone on the ward. It made the very frequent lavatorial trips so much easier to take.

The single room was a great advantage not just for me, but I would think that all of the patients share this viewpoint. I found that the preservation of dignity was very important and being private helped this tremendously. The tabloids carry stories of patients in mixed sex wards of 20 people and call the practice disgraceful and degrading. It is not often that I agree with the tabloids, but on this point they are absolutely right. My room was sparse, which helps to keep infection down, but had sufficient room for the bed, drip stands, T. V. visitors chairs, and a Recliner if you were lucky as I was. A door opened on to a toilet and shower, during the period of diuretics, the door hinges almost had metal fatigue. Outside was an exercise bike, a sink for visitors use, altogether a compact, functional unit.

The only disadvantage was that it tended to make life a bit solitary. It was awkward in any case talking to other patients, as there was always a risk of infection, and we tended not to talk very much, which was a shame.

During the early stages, nothing seemed to be happening. I had a slight tight feeling between my eyes during the anti-emetic treatment, otherwise nothing. The physiotherapist called and gave me an exercise regime which seemed to be extremely untaxing, and would do nothing to lessen my steroid driven ballooning weight. I was horrified at being 13st 10, but the nurses insisted that I should make no effort to reduce weight. They obviously knew what was likely to happen, and I was not astute enough to pick it up.

The day drifted on, a glorious spring day, and as my room overlooked the open country, at least the view was pleasant. Had my T. V. been working it may have been more interesting, but my pump developed a fault which was more annoying. The pump, as the name implies gets the fluids and Chemotherapy into my body, and is designed so that a battery takes over when the electricity is disconnected, enabling the whole unit to be trundled into the toilet. On occasions the pump would not restart, when the mains electricity was reconnected and a nurse had to come and reset it. None of them gave the slightest sign of annoyance, but it must have been a complete waste of time correcting faulty equipment.

News from the great wide world outside, Sunderland have won again, providing a boost for patients everywhere (apart from Newcastle). Kenny Everett has died. Although I have no time for his life style, he was a genuinely inventive and funny man, which is not a bad trait in a comedian. He paid no lip service at all to political correctness, these modern trends are set to drive us all mad. A cancer patient has been denied treatment at Addenbrooke's and the media is in full swing.

This is what I find disgraceful about some sections of the press and T.V. The poor girl known only as Child B was refused further treatment as the hospital did not think she had a good chance of recovery, and that it was not in her best interests. This was no good for the press who thought a much better story would be if she was refused treatment on financial grounds, and that is how they ran it. The fact that at the same meeting in which funds were refused for "Child B "another treatment was approved which was far more expensive, but had a very good chance of success was never mentioned. This is a good journalistic principle, never let the facts get in the way of a good story.

The only good thing about the publicity is that a private clinic have offered to try an experimental treatment. I hope this is a genuine attempt and not offered for financial reasons. When I hear of children being seriously ill, I feel awful. I would love to see her cheat the quoted survival odds of 10 to 1, even though she may have a rough ride.

5 April 1995

I had a bad night last night. When I lay down, I felt bloated and slightly nauseous, which could be due to the phenomenal amounts of fluid I am taking. The real problem is that every time I go for a pee, the pump alarms, and one of the nurses has to come and reset the thing. It is only the second day and already it is irritating me. I managed a little breakfast, but it was a struggle. June thinks that I should eat as much as possible, but on one of the very rare occasions I will go against her advice. Eating is getting to be a chore, most unusual for me.

The nurses are collecting my specimens to measure the intake and output to make sure I was taking enough fluid to protect my liver and kidneys. Steroids make me constipated so there was no sign of a specimen for the girls to collect. Strange thing to collect, but I suppose it is much the same as train numbers for excitement. The agenda for today is one bag of fluid, one 3 hour chemo, and off the pump for the rest of the day.

Observations, temperature, blood pressure and pulse are taken regularly , and the doctors make regular visits. On one visit Isobel looked in my mouth and was very interested in the hard lumps I have at the base of my teeth. She seemed very relieved when I told her that I had had them for as long as I could remember. My dentist has a fancy name for them, but they are not doing any harm, and as long as that persists, we will leave well alone.

Lunch was served, and for the first time in my life, I could not finish it. June was due at around 2 o'clock, with Chris and Barry to follow I settled down to watch T.V.; it must have donated by the Ecology party, it was completely green, and totally useless. By this time I was used to the routine visits from the nurses doing observations, collecting bottles, etc., but they seemed to be coming more often for a chat, almost as if they were watching for something . They were.

I had to be sick during visiting which was a bit inconvenient, but unavoidable. The sister stayed in the room for a while, I assumed to talk to June and get to know her. Looking back the real reason was probably more prosaic. If I was to get a reaction to the chemo, it would come about now. I had just finished telling the nurses that I felt fine, and my cockiness was destroyed in one fell swoop.

It started with a red face, bad headache, jaw and teeth aching, stiff neck, and an inability to keep my legs and arms still. I was given drugs straight into my line, and it did nothing for the pain for what seemed like hours. Just as it looked like a mallet was the next step, the drugs took hold, and slowly, very slowly the pain receded. By the time June went home at about 7, things were not too bad, and I was able to pretend that I was better than I was. I would hate June to go home thinking I was still in pain. I was unable to eat anything which was incredible for me, and gradually drifted off to sleep.

It had been a bad, bad, day

6 April 1995

I slept the sleep of the drugged, did not wake up apart from the observations, and felt much better. I am determined to keep up exercise as long as I can and had a bike ride for 15 minutes, and a walk round the ward. My determination to carry on as normal I felt to be important. I made up my mind that no matter how I felt, I would always shower and get dressed. I had noticed patients still in dressing gowns in the afternoons, and I had the theory that I would feel better if I carried on as near to normal as possible.

In order to take the next batch of chemo, I need to be passing 500 ml per hour. Converted to pounds shillings and pence, this is nearly a pint, and I was concerned that my output would be insufficient for the next chemo to begin. The treatment is so strong that it needs to be washed through with fluid, or kidney damage is possible. In the event my fears were groundless, I passed (yes passed) with flying colours, it could have something to do with the fact that I was taking in 1000ml through the line. No need for any Abbot Ale, and the chemo started on time which was important as the schedule was tight.

No problems occurred with the last chemo, it is all in, and no sign of any sickness which is a noted side effect. My appetite is getting worse. It could be due to a sore mouth, or hospital food, or my taste buds altering but it is having an effect. My long awaited specimen has at last arrived, and I have given it to the girl who collects them. A lovely girl, but she has strange hobbies.

I had a talk to Paul who is the only male nurse on C10. He gave me an update on how things were going, and we seem to have no problems. The last test showed the myeloma cells were down to 5%, before my last chemo was on board. He thought that I would have 5 rough days next week, but possibly go home in 14 days. It seems that my bone marrow is now almost dead, and that I am now reliant on the stem cells which were harvested some 2 weeks ago. It is a good job I have total confidence in the hospital, this is no time for mixing labels up or losing bags of stem cells. Apparently it looks like smoked salmon, I hope they can tell the difference.

News from outside is that Swindon lost and as they are in the relegation zone with Sunderland it has to be good news. Everything is coming good I am starting to recover a bit of my bounce.

I settle down to bed a lot happier, bottles notwithstanding, and look forward to the big day tomorrow. Friday is transplant day.

Chapter Three –
Into The Valley Of The Transplant

Day 4 Friday. Day 0

Transplant day is always described as 0, subsequent days are 0+1, 0+2, and so on. The transplant is to take place at 2 this afternoon, and the morning passed well. I now have my T.V. and Video, June is bringing a CD player when she comes. Already I am a typical patient, watching the clock for visitors. Although visitors can come at any time, we feel it would disturb the ward routine if we told people that, so we stick to the afternoon. June normally comes at 2 and I miss her so much, if she is ever late, it is awful. She has other problems apart from me. Sue, the sister on her ward is ill, and even in my ignorance it sounds very serious. This means that June has to run the ward, as well as visit me, it must be a tremendous strain.

I had the last fluids during the morning, but I am finding it progressively difficult to eat. When we were married I was 9st 5, and unless I start to eat soon, I will be heading for that again. In my present drug bloated condition, I am well over 13st, but I have been told that it will not last. I can still get out for exercise, but the way my blood counts are falling, it will not be for long. There are many dangers: infection when the white cells are low and internal bruising when the platelets are low. My white cells are plummeting and it is stupid to take risks.

This whole operation has been in preparation for the transplant. The chemo has killed the bone marrow, hence the falling counts, and the stem cells which have been cultured and purified are ready to be collected. Come to think of it, when the cultured cells are in my body, it will be the only part of me that is cultured. Leading up to 2 o'clock was a sense of anticipation, and as the time got near, I was expecting a fanfare, or a roll of drums, or at the very least, lots of people in green gowns and wellies. Not a bit of it, it was a complete anticlimax.

My cells came in a bag, with a small amount of clear liquid in, which was unceremoniously attached to my trusty line and that was that. I did notice my name written clearly on the bag, as this is the only danger in the procedure up to now. I have no immune system at all, and am totally reliant on the transplant working, at least it is a good start if they have the right cells. It was all over in 20 minutes, and I was left with a strange smell of sweetcorn, and was thankful of a supply of boiled sweets. The smell was strong, as I went down in the lift for one of my last walks, everyone was asking what the smell was.

I only said "It is me", leaving it for June to expand a little, but the people in the lift probably had a good idea anyway. The chemo boys are easy to spot. They wear caps and although there are many middle age men who are bald, they have eyebrows and eyelashes, chemo boys have neither. Also, C10 is at the top of the hospital therefore anyone staying in the lift is likely to have a transplant so there is no hiding where the sweetcorn smell is coming from. Strange thing is the lift tends to empty before the top floors. Presumably those requiring the Genito ward get off at the floor below and walk up.

So apart from transfusions of blood or platelets, it is all over, I am simply waiting for my counts to come up, and I can go home. There is a great danger of infections now, but I was surprised to find that it was not from outsiders, but from within me that the infections would come. I have told the nurses that I will the first patient to go through without an infection, let us see if cockiness can baffle bugs. In layman's logic, the chemo has wiped out everything in my bone marrow, including the myeloma cells. The stem cells have been purified and transplanted back, and as they are my own cells there is no problem of rejection. It only needs the cells to grow, and replace the immune system and I am cured. All so simple really.

Saturday Day 5. Day plus 1

This has been a good day, apart from the smell of sweet corn or asparagus which is still hanging around me. Paul (the male nurse not the son) took me through the progress so far, and it looks good to me. After 3 doses of chemo through my portable pump, the cancer cells were less than 5%. Since then I have had another cassette chemo, and all the drips here, so I can not see much being left. The stitches have come out of my line, and Paul thinks they can be left rather than being re-done which is another bonus. Paul is a really nice bloke, and like everyone else here, any questions are answered calmly and factually which suits me fine.

My appetite and taste buds continue to give me problems. It is less a case of small appetite than outright revulsion. Apart from this there is a tightness between my eyes, and the continuing constipation due to the damned steroids. I feel a personal hatred towards the steroids, I just hope they are doing some good to counteract the rotten feeling they cause.

I ended with a load of visitors. June came with Ian (No 1 son), and Barry and Chris called later. It being Grand National day we spent a few minutes picking the prospective winners. Barry and Chris both won, the least said about our efforts the better. Also, Sunderland beat Derby away, we will escape relegation yet.

Just a thought. I am depending on the stem cells colonising my bone marrow and producing healthy cells. How do they know where to swim? I hope mine are not thick, or land lubbers.

Sunday Day 6. 0 plus 2

Pretty uneventful, the usual vile taste in my mouth, appetite still getting less. I had a bad nights sleep which does not help much, and with the hated steroids on top, I am feeling a bit down. Part of it is that I am missing June and being at home. I had better be careful or I will end up being depressed. It is through no fault of the Ward but I feel lonely at times and find it hard to relax. The nurses come in and out and are very welcome, but it is not like being at home.

My counts have not reached rock bottom yet, so I was able to go out, and had a walk round the hospital grounds. I am clearly not as strong as I was, but I took it gently and managed reasonably well. I am pioneering an idea the hospital have, which seems logical to me. They say that every patient gets some form of infection, and rather then waiting for it to happen, they put an injection into my line which it is hoped will prevent it occurring.

From the world of sport, I was pleased to see Damon Hill win, and Tottenham lose. They used to be one of my favourite non-Sunderland teams but they have let themselves down badly over the illegal payments fiasco. Over recent years Peterborough were relegated, as were Swindon, and their transgressions were less serious than Tottenham. The difference is that Tottenham have lots of clout with the F.A, and lots of money to fight legal battles, and they ended up with a smacked wrist.

I suppose it could be my magistrates training which makes me hate injustice, or it could be that my hatred of injustice led me to become a magistrate.

Monday Day 7. 0 plus 3

Still able to walk outside the hospital, not being as yet neutropaedic, which is the state of having no immune system. I managed my walk, but was noticeably slower than yesterday. My counts are very low, but not yet low enough to keep me indoors. The steroids have stopped, and therefore my constipation has eased, and I am able to produce stool specimens. Tracey was once more on duty when the collection was made, it happens every time. I hope that she doesn't do the pools, with her luck she will get nowhere.

I have noticed that every nurse and doctor look in my mouth, they are obviously expecting one of the side effects to manifest itself. Problems could be in the mouth itself, or the throat or gullet, or all three. On top of that stomach cramps could be a problem, and the medics are clearly expecting it to start soon. Hopefully this means that the sooner the problem is spotted, the sooner it can be dealt with.

A pleasant surprise, Graham Honeywood called. It was nice to see him, and I was feeling all right, so I could talk to him. All the years we have known each other, and I hadn't a clue his office was in Cambridge. After he left, I tried to eat, but failed miserably. Unless anyone has been through this, it is impossible to relate just how awful it is, made all the worse for me as my appetite previously was so good. It would be unfair to say that I went hungry as a child, but with my love of sport I was always active and have always had a tremendous appetite. It was clear however that money was very tight, and there was no food to waste. I got into the habit of clearing my plate on every occasion, and it mattered not if I had the same dish over and over again. Even in the Forces, nothing escaped back into the kitchen. They used to say in the R.A.F that they will have to start spelling gannet with two n's and two t's. What a contrast between then and now, and it is getting worse.

So we sit tight and wait for the bone marrow to crash, and the side effects to start. There is a catalogue of drugs to help me once it happens, but I feel that it is coming, and the rough times may not be far off. I just have to sit without an immune system for a few days until my stem cells start growing. I had assumed that Ward C10 was at the top of the hospital for reasons of infection, and that there would be a higher air pressure in the ward than outside. This would prevent air borne infections from coming in. It seems that I was wrong, we are at the top of the hospital by chance, and no one knows of any pressure system, so it seems that I am giving them credit to which they are not due. So I sit waiting either for my immune system to pick up, or an infection to start, and I hope that it is the right order. Timing is of the essence.

Tuesday Day 8. 0 plus 4

My counts are almost at the bottom, my immune system is virtually nonexistent. Because of this, my license has been withdrawn and I can no longer leave the ward. Also I am banned from using the exercise bike. I must not bruise myself, and although I would have thought that a bruise was minor, this is different. A bruise could cause internal bleeding, a crack on the head could cause cranial bleeding and this was a good reason for me to behave myself. It seems that the low point is coming, but there is a good factor about that. The sooner the low point is reached, the sooner I will start to improve, and go home.

Probably the side effects will rear up shortly, I am certainly a lot more tired, I walk up and down the corridor, and I feel is if I have divers boots on. It certainly does not help my appetite, I am now eating almost nothing, and I am becoming quite concerned. The trick is to keep up to as near full strength as possible, eating nothing is not helping. I survive on semi liquid food, and if it carries on for long, I will be revolted by the gloop I am forcing down and end up with nothing.

I had loads of visitors today, June of course, but also Bert, Janet, Muriel and Peter. Peter was diagnosed with Motor Neurone Disease almost two years ago, and he is an absolute inspiration. Compared to Peter's illness mine is a cakewalk, and yet he still drives, plays golf and walks every day. He is remarkable. I have read in the past where famous people have been struck down with this, and they seem to last a very short while. David Niven and Don Revie seemed to be a lot less well than Peter, it would not surprise me if he was the first to recover from it.

I had a needless worry earlier. A large filling dropped out, and my first thought was that if any extraction or drilling was necessary, with my low platelets, I might be in trouble. In the event, the decision was that unless it was bothering me, to leave well alone. This suited me fine, I am always prepared to listen to reasons why I should not go to the dentist. Ordinarily, it would have been a problem with food getting into the cavity, but at least I was spared that with my absence of eating. Every cloud has a silver lining.

A few minutes of farce followed when the visitors left. I am glad that they came on a reasonably good day, and although it tires me, it is great to see them. One of the nurses mentioned that my sore mouth would be helped by gargling. At this point I realised that my life so far had not taught me anything useful, in short, I had no idea how to. The nurse gave some general advice, and left. She came back in a short while, and had better advice, obviously she had no idea either, and had been to ask somebody. Gargling is a strange concept, but I will have a try.

Wednesday Day 9. 0 plus 5

My mouth is becoming troublesome, it is very sore, and it feels thick, I hope my hamfisted efforts at gargling are helping. I can still manage a few trips up and down the corridor, the lap count was 15, but I felt very tired. My blood counts are obviously low, and I am having a blood transfusion later. In my time as a blood donor, I gave 79 pints, so I am now getting a bit of my own back.

I am now being sick at odd times, but this has nothing to do with food, as I can now not face anything. In the morning, Pat left the menu in my room, and I was sick immediately. By the afternoon, I could not think of water without feeling sick. I couldn't have caught Rabies could I? The dietician called, and put me on a liquid diet, and said that if the worst happened, I could be fed through my line. The only thing I can take is milk and as long as I can take it, I should keep going until I can eat again.

Barry and Chris came, and quite stupidly, I tried to stay awake and join in the conversation. I should have had the sense to sleep. I cannot be bothered with T.V. or books and cannot remember a time when I slept so much. My inclination is to pretend I am better than I am, but this is crazy, making me tired, and in any case my contribution to the conversation is about four or five grunts. My attitude is not backed up by much logic I am afraid, but I sometimes think that if I admit that I am not well that I am giving in. Illogical it may be, but thoughts like these do intrude from time to time.

By the evening, I could not pretend any longer, odd rashes were appearing on my body. I wondered if this was with all the milk I was drinking, must remember to ask June if babies get rashes. I was sick again, the observations showed that my temperature was rising, and it felt like as the temperature rose, my spirits fell. I had told the nurses that I would be the first patient to go through without an infection. They said that the chances were remote, and as usual it looks like they are going to be right.

Thursday Day 10. 0 plus 6

It has been a pretty awful day, and at the moment seems to be getting worse. Even though I am on a liquid diet, I am still being sick. I hope that doesn't mean feeding through the line. However daft, I will feel that I have failed if we have to resort to that. The tablets appear to be making me sick, and I am now bringing up blood.

At least I got the problems out of the way before the visitors arrived. Pat and Ken are really good company, even better if we were all in their house or mine. When they left I was tired and virtually went straight to sleep. I find it so comforting when June is there even if I can't speak much. It is very difficult to stay awake for any length of time, and even harder to put on a front when June calls.

I think I am feeling sorry for myself, as long as no one is overly sympathetic I should be all right.

Friday Day 11. 0 plus 7

Today has been a slight improvement, I am taking fluids, and not being sick as much. Blood is still coming out of my mouth which could be the level of platelets, now reading 6. Also I am starting with heartburn which is uncomfortable.

I am writing these notes late at night as I have little recollection of being awake today. Ian called and I was asleep for a good 50% of the time, doubly annoying as he brings me the football news. One thing Addenbrooke's lacks is a T.V. with Ceefax. When June was here my sleep rate must have been 90%. Although I am still sticking to my target of dressing and showering every day, I only move from bed to my recliner and go to sleep there.

I must be in the running for the Rip Van Winkle award.

Saturday Day 12. 0 plus 8

My notes are getting less, and more difficult to read. I am awake less, and too exhausted to remember much, and it is all a bit of a shambles. I needed a chest x-ray, and I was taken down in my bed clutching my little bottle in case my reservoir flooded, and the way they took me was totally different to the public corridors. It is a different world off the beaten track.

June arrived just as I got back, and suggested that she should stop Jim and Judy coming. I agreed with sadness, as it would be the first time I could not face people. I may have made the effort, but I knew that Jim finds hospitals and illness hard to take, so we advised them not to come. This deprived them of my scintillating grunts, but could not be helped. Jim, like Ken is Irish and they are both tremendous company. They have a different sense of humour and are great fun, particularly when aided by alcohol.

My temperature is a little higher, but in line with the expected level, so nothing to worry about. If things go as they are, I might need a painkiller overnight. It seems crazy in a place like this, but I still do not like taking drugs.

Sunderland drew at home, another welcome point.

Sunday Day 13. 0 plus 9

Very vague day, I can recall very little. I was told that I was complaining of heartburn, and had more platelets injected but have no recollection. I was desperately tired and have vague memories of people coming in and out and talking about stitching my line in again. As long as they only talk about it I fear not.

I am now coming into a phase which I was told to expect and which I was dreading, the onset of diarrhoea. Up to now as I have mentioned, I have had nothing to do with hospitals, and now I had to put up with diarrhoea so bad that I didn't know when it was happening. My worst time was during the night when I think I got through six pairs of pyjamas. The girls came and sorted me out without a trace of annoyance or reproach. If they had done so, I would have felt ashamed and humiliated. They saved me all of that, they were wonderful.

The dreaded re-stitching of my line happened after all. I was just dozing off at night when the Casualty Officer came up and did the deed. As with most things, the anticipation is worse than the event, and I hardly knew what she was doing. We were chatting about something or other which took my mind off what she was doing and it was no problem at all.

Monday Day 14. 0 plus 10

I scribbled a few lines of notes today and am now totally unable to decipher them. My mind was wandering in and out of sanity. Ian and June were here, and I never knew. Looking at my scribblings I will need to combine a few days together, and decipher as much as I can of the hallucinations. It is possible with a bit of goodwill to recognise it as attempted writing but apart from the odd word or two it is gibberish.

Tuesday Day 15. 0 plus 11

This has been an awful day, certainly the worst yet. Temperature over 100°F, this is the way I have always thought of temperature. Anything over 100 is bad, and it certainly is. I could tell when I came back from a "trip" that I must have been gibbering by the looks on the faces of the people in the room. Only twice, I woke up and people who had been in my hallucination were actually in the room, and this threw me for a few seconds until I realised what was going on. This is what madness must be like, and it is a very disturbing experience and not one which I ever want to repeat.

Gradually throughout the day, my temperature started to come down, and I started to have more blood transfusions. My levels have started to improve, and Dr. Marcus thinks I should bounce back now. I am still unable to take tablets, or drink properly, and am totally exhausted. Visitors came and went and I am sorry indeed for the harrowing time they must have had. I still in some way feel guilty when I am not able to entertain visitors, crazy though it is; that is what I feel.

All round, and in every way, it has been a bad, bad ,day.

Wednesday 16 April. day 0 plus 12
Thursday 17 April. day 0 plus 13
Friday 18 April. day 0 plus 14

I had resolved to scribble a few notes down each night, but for these three days, not even indecipherable scrawl was possible. One day I tried to scribble something down, but it is just possible to tell that it is an attempt at writing certainly no chance of reading it. I had no idea of night and day, but slipped in and out of sleep and therefore having no idea when night was, I could be excused for not writing notes at night.

I have looked at a copy of my attempt at writing notes at sometime during this period, and even now, it is very difficult to pick out more than the odd word.

The odd gap has been filled in by things that Dr Marcus or June have said, but it is all a vague nonsense from my point of view. Alf and Eileen called after driving all the way from Newcastle. Whilst I have always thought that leaving Newcastle must always be an improvement, it is an awful long way to come and watch me sleeping, moaning, and twitching.

It is very hard to remember the content of my hallucinations, which is logical. If I could remember them in detail, I wouldn't have been having them. From what I have pieced together, it involved a drugs ring operating through the Mafia, and delivering supplies to a factory complex. The name of the complex was the same as a building contractor who has a hoarding on the way to Cambridge, so that can be explained.

What is more difficult is what was going on. I know that my eldest son was involved along with two of the nurses, but they must have been the good guys for they seemed to be keeping watch. The complex has a circular dome, and when supplies arrived a section of the wall slid up, and came down immediately, giving no chance for anyone to gain access, or see inside. These very small recollections are all I can remember, similar to waking up after a dream. I suspect that the hallucinations were very unpleasant, as I usually felt really awful when I came round, perhaps there is a body mechanism which shuts the memory banks down when required. So this is really all I can say about my missing days, perhaps it is just as well.

Saturday Day 19. 0 plus 15

I thought of a terrible old joke which could be modified to this situation. "How many F's in Platelets?" There is no F in Platelets. That's what we have been telling you". My platelet count is still low, the others are fine. One theory is that the anti-biotics I am taking are wiping out my platelets and hence no growth. It will have to be sorted out if I am to be discharged. To let me out before my immune system is working would be like having me as a germ magnet. My throat and mouth are still sore, apparently the lining disintegrates with the ravages of the chemo, as does the stomach lining and the gut. No wonder eating is such an ordeal.

On the Australian front, Andie and Steve have sent a terrific newspaper front page. The story is standard, but the headline can be anything under the sun. I have the page on my wall, proclaiming "Ray Grummett signs for Sunderland", and it is admired by all. I missed out in my footballing days as although I was fit, dead keen and dedicated, I had not a shred of talent. The other great thing from Australia is from Paul (No 2 son) who is in Australia having a year off before completing his degree. He is depicted on a card, sitting in his Sunderland strip, talking to the Pope, who is praying. The caption reads "Carry on John, we need the points".

The news has just been on T.V. Sunderland won again, God bless Peter Reid, and now we need only one point to stay up. Surely, lads, surely you can manage that for me.

Sunday Day 20. 0 plus 16

I now feel as if I have this thing on the run. I feel fine except for obvious things like lack of sleep. My observations are now hourly, so clearly sleep is curtailed. The diarrhoea is still troublesome, but manageable. Apart from this, I feel fine, honestly. I admit that I always say that I am feeling fine, it is an automatic response from one who would hate to be considered a whinger. It fooled only me, however, I heard Dr. Marcus ask June one day, "Is he really all right?"

In a misplaced fit of euphoria, I asked for a bacon sandwich, but after a tiny bite, put it away. I may have solved one problem, though, of why even the bread tastes horrible. It looks very much like that Mighty White, and that is enough to put anyone off.

I am being continually assessed, X Rays, etc., and if I can drink 1 litre of fluid per day, I need not have any through the line. Having fluids through the line is no big deal, but I want to get back to normality. I want to get rid of all lines and tubes quickly, and have my case heard before the escape committee.

I feel fine, I believe I am well, but the drugs I am taking are making me ill, the fluids are making me ill, the lack of sleep is making me ill, and the lack of food is making me ill. At some stage, we have to listen to my body, and I am sure I am right. A bit of home cooking, and a pint of Abbot, and I will be transformed.

Monday Day 21. 0 plus 17

Probably my best day yet. True there are a few problems still like sore and puffy eyes, fingers bleeding as the skin falls off, and the skin rashes are taking a while to go away. Also, I have nose bleeds, and my nurse tells me not to adopt the normal masculine solution for anything nasal. What she means is keep your fingers to yourself. I would not dream of naming her as all the nurses have been great, but if I had to pick a favourite she would be it.

When I was having all the fluids and drugs, this particular nurse was on duty. I found out that it was safer to have the arms on top of the drip lines, as if they were underneath, they could be torn out during sleep. As I had two lines, I crossed my arms over my chest and dozed off. I heard my nurse say "Ray, we don't like people to lie like that in here". It might be classed as black humour, but what a tonic a sense of humour is.

I am now simply waiting for the Doctors to let me go home. My bad patch is over, I have been through the mill, and am now out the other side. All tubes are out, and all drugs are stopped. It seems that I have had a bad reaction to two of the drugs, otherwise everything is fine. I have seen two different teams of doctors today, one group says I should be out on Wednesday, the other on Friday, we are saying Saturday, anything earlier is a bonus.

Now that I can enjoy visitors again, I have had Barry and Chris in the morning, and Judy and Jim in the afternoon. Very good company and a tonic. I still have a sore mouth and throat but have developed into a fair little gargler. What a talent this boy has.

Tuesday Day 22. 0 plus 18

I am still trying to force food down with very little success. This obviously is the reason why I was told to ignore my bloated weight when I came in as it is melting away now. Whilst walking round the corridors, I saw a group of youngsters about 19-21 relaxing on the grass presumably having a break from lectures. I remembered myself at that age, in the R.A.F. and superbly fit, glowing with health and vigour. What a pale husk of that man I have become.

The doctors called again and I ended up with more platelets, and this is the only problem now, they are not growing quickly enough. My resistance is so poor that I am vulnerable to anything I come into contact with. At that point one of my sisters thought she would visit me and bring the grandchildren with her. This would have been like a time bomb for me and I was relieved when she decided to wait until I was at home.

Wednesday Day 23. 0 plus 19

I feel stronger and seem to be sleeping better, although my mouth is still very dry. I am on nursing only now, just the usual observations, and the specimen collections for weighing and testing. I felt good, and was unprepared for an assessment of my platelet problem which knocked me sideways.

The doctors now think that my immune system is regarding the new platelets as aliens and are destroying them but that it may be temporary. May be, what does that mean? Do I have to spend the rest of my days here? How long will the rest of my days be? If I am to be allowed home, the options seem to be:

1) to go to Harlow for platelet transfusions.

2) to wait for the platelets to put themselves right.

To be fair, the doctors did not seem concerned, but it shook the hell out of me. In trying to see some good in all of this, it surely means that my white cells are working well. If they are destroying the platelets they must be strong enough to cope with normal infections.

In telling me of the possibility of my platelets being cannibalised in this way the doctors disturbed me. Good doctors they may be, but I don't think much of their P.R. The Sister, Terri must have noticed my reaction and called back a few minutes later to put my mind at rest. It may seem only a small thing but it had a disproportionate effect. Bless you Terri.

Wednesday 26 April.

I was released on "License", meaning that I can be recalled at any time if the counts are poor. There will still be a need to go back to the Evelyn for platelets on alternate days which involves a lot of travelling but it is great to be home. I have a list of foods to avoid for different reasons. Hot curries would irritate my stomach, anything salty would irritate my mouth and throat. Foods containing raw ingredients, like Steak Tartare, Mayonnaise and all salads are banned together with anything not cooked thoroughly in case of infection. I can drink in moderation, but not real ale which has an active ingredient, yeast. Spirits are all banned for the time being as again, this would act as an irritant. It will be something to look forward to but my bottle of Isle of Jura must stay hidden away for now. What may have been a problem for others is much less so for me as sadly I am eating so little that I will not need to deprive myself of very much at all. Chilli con carne is some way in the distance.

Chapter Four – The First Come Back

Tuesday 2 May

It may be great to be home again but I am staggered at my weakness. Any effort at all and I am so tired that I doze off wherever I am. Weakness is a relative word. An athlete would be weak if he could only manage a mile in 4 minutes 10 seconds. My definition of weakness is not being able to lift a kettle with one hand, that is my kind of weakness. One day Eira called, a colleague from Dow Stoker, and I made her a cup of coffee. By the time she left I was so tired and weak that I was unable to carry the cups back into the kitchen. Dr Marcus said that I had to stay out of the garden for a while in case of infection. I can see the point in that, but the real reason I stay out of the garden is that I am afraid a caterpillar will grab me and cart me off to its lair.

I am still unable to eat, a great disappointment, as I was hoping that it was hospital food that was holding me back. No such luck. The vile taste in my mouth carries on and the appetite which only a couple of months ago was a force to be reckoned with is now almost extinct. My first attempt at eating was a disaster. I tried a tiny piece of fish and vomited immediately. Even the smell of food is revolting and I have decided to have my morsels in the living room out of the way of the cooking smells.

Wednesday 3 May

Quite without warning my temperature shot up to 38.5°C, which equates to 100°F plus. The standing instructions are to get back to Addenbrooke's sharpish and a quick decision had to be made. As we live 45 minutes from the hospital we could not afford to take a chance, and consequently with heavy heart, packed a bag and off we went. It is a delicate balancing act when the temperature shoots up like this. I could assume that is an aberration and stay at home and see what happens, which is always my choice. The problem is that if I wait too long by the time I finally arrive at the hospital what was a problem may well be a crisis.

It was nearly midnight when we arrived and I was worried about June driving back on her own at this time of night. I need not have worried the nurses had arranged a bed for June without being asked. It is actions like that which make Addenbrooke's such a good place to be. In the event they put my temperature down to reaction from the platelets and it was back to 36.5° which is my normal by morning.

Thursday 4 May

When I last saw Dr Marcus he said that with luck I could be back to work in a month. I didn't say much, but I know how I feel and to meet this time scale a tremendous improvement is needed. Still he has seen it all before, let us hope he is right.

Friday 5 May

I will keep this to myself for now, but this morning, I could tell the difference between mouth wash and toothpaste. The vile taste is still there, and I have no wish to eat, so I will not raise hopes about a comeback just yet. Still, it proves that something is happening and the aversion to food may be the next thing to be beaten.

Saturday 6 May

Had more platelets, and noticed a slight rise in temperature, but not enough to worry about. My low platelets problem is still with us, and this week may be the crunch time. My problem seems to be that –

1) I am not producing sufficient platelets, or

2) I am producing plenty, but my immune system is destroying them which is what one of the Addenbrooke's doctors said.

The difference was that Dr Marcus said that whichever of the options it turns out to be, it can be corrected. This piece of information was omitted before and if I had known this I would not have been as concerned. If nothing happens this week I will need to go back to the Evelyn for another biopsy, which hopefully will sort it out one way or the other.

Things are not going as smooth as I had hoped but then nobody said it would be easy.

Tuesday 9 May

June thinks I am losing my fight. She may be right; she usually is. My eyes are dull and lifeless and this is a useful barometer for me. Many years ago a girl said to me that I had lovely eyes, "like a spaniel in pain". I wonder what she would think now. If the eyes are the window of the soul I wonder how this leaves me as my eyes are like a filthy toilet window in a railway station.

It is true, though, that although I have not consciously given up, I feel totally lethargic and lacking in spirit. The problems as I see them are –

(1) The slow improvement causing frustration.

(2) My hopeless food intake.

(3) My platelet problem.

I want to go on to a liquid diet to save me the terrible anguish of facing food. Every one is opposed to this idea but clever as Dr Marcus and the nurses (including June in this) are, the only people who truly know what it is like is another chemo patient.

I go to the Evelyn tomorrow, and I trust Dr Marcus will tell me in a clear and straightforward way how he wants to proceed, this is his style. It is just a nagging fear that if my immune system has turned rogue and can't be corrected where does that leave me? A good pointer is that Dr Marcus wants to take my line out and he wouldn't be thinking of that if he knew that lots of platelet or blood transfusions would be needed.

Whatever it takes, let us get it sorted out.

Wednesday 10 May

Once or twice I have felt that my taste was altering, but it was difficult to be sure because of the vile taste in my mouth. I went back to the Evelyn for a bone marrow aspiration, my third. They seem to get worse, perhaps I know what is coming, and the anticipation is worse than the actual. During the examination, Dr Marcus noticed thrush in my mouth and I was annoyed with myself for not realising this sooner. The nasty taste, slimy sensation, and nasty deposits should have alerted me. I had only ever heard of babies and women getting thrush and I was pleasantly surprised when I did not have to fend off any disreputable questions from my friends. Talking of friends, they are proving to be invaluable. The times when June has to go to work could be lonely, but hardly a day goes by without someone calling. Barry and Bert share my love of football and it was good to have them call for a chat even though my contribution was sometimes less than sparkling. David Watts called, another colleague who had learned from Eira that I was well enough to have visitors, it was great to see him.

Be that as it may I am back on the tablets, and if nothing else, curing the thrush should make me feel better. I had more platelets and by Friday we should be able to tell how they are doing. Also, and more importantly for me, the lab will be able to count the remaining myeloma cells. My money is on nil, I would hate to have come all this way for nothing.

Friday 12 May

I have a feeling that things are improving. The mouth still tastes awful, I am as weak as the proverbial kitten, but the bone marrow test showed that I am producing loads of platelets. My own body defences are wiping the new cells out unfortunately, and just as bad is the classic cure for this problem – steroids. I hate taking them, but needs must.

The great news is that my prediction was correct, the myeloma cell count is nil. To a layman this means that I am cured, but of course Dr Marcus is more cautious and rightly so. The test showed that there were no myeloma cells in the batch tested but it is still possible that the odd one may still be lurking around. He did, however, call it extremely encouraging so I am happy to settle for that.

Just let me get back to eating and get my comeback on course.

Saturday 13 May

I am eating small amounts as one of the effects of steroids is an increase in appetite. The taste sensation is still appalling, but small things are happening. Today I found that Lasagne tastes different to banana, so there is hope for me yet. I have also been able to keep warm for the first time since leaving hospital.

This may have been coincidence, but our cat came back to me. Since I got our of hospital he has had nothing to do with me and it has been absurd watching this great bruiser of a cat trying to fit onto June's very small lap. Anyway, he decided that this day he would return, and went to sleep quite happily. I like cats, particularly this one, but they are completely selfish creatures and their own comfort is paramount. He wouldn't have come back to me unless he felt it was right. Animals seem to have a sixth sense about people who are ill. When our dog was with us he always sat very close to my mother, perhaps it was his instinct being a sheep dog.

Monday 15 May

I seem to be improving. I feel stronger. I can stand up from a chair which previously I would have had to lever myself up from. My waking times are getting longer and my food intake is still tiny, but not now minuscule. I am constantly looking for good signs, and I think my hair may be coming back which is important. Dr Marcus has an adage, "when your hair is back, you are back". The slight down side is that along with hair growth comes beard growth, but beggars can't be choosers.

One great occasion I had my first walk outside and was amazed at how uneven pavements are it took some concentration to stay upright. Also, with June's help, I had a small walk in the garden and it is a terrific landmark. Surely I am on the comeback trail.

Wednesday 17 May

I am improving but so gradually that it is hard to be certain. My appetite is still very poor and still I have the awful taste in my mouth. I should consider going to the dentist but that is only slightly better than more chemo.

My beard is definitely starting to grow again along with the other tufts of hair. Shaving is a nuisance but it is a concrete sign that things are returning to normal. It will be nice to have eyelashes and eyebrows again. People look at me and wonder what it is about me that is strange it takes a chemo man to know another. I have never been troubled with vanity but I had given no thought that it would include all hair, not just the head. Bath times reminded me of the last chicken in Sainsbury's for quite some time. During the time my hair has been missing, a few people have called me Kojak, which is not so bad. Uncle Fester I am not so sure about.

I went to the dentist, and thanks to Roger Beeching it was not in any way an ordeal. I had problems with transport, with waiting around, and was a bit afraid of coming into contact with the general public for fear of infection. Roger solved everything under the old pals act, having been friends for 20 years. One evening he called, took me to his Surgery at about 7, when all the other patients had gone, did the filling and took me home again. No fear of infection, in fact no fear at all, which is unusual for me. Bless you Roger, you certainly did me proud.

Sunday 21 May

Six days ago, I took my first uncertain steps outside. Now I routinely go round the block (1/4 mile), or round the block via the main road (1/2 mile), and today I went down to the village for the first time. I was quite proud of myself, and although I was tired, was not exhausted. My friends have all offered to accompany me on these walks, but I would rather do it on my own. There is the sense of achievement, and also less risk of boring themselves silly at the speed I go. They still call to see me at home and I enjoy their company and look forward to them coming. Sometimes up to four call at once, and although the banter tires me, I can always sleep afterwards, and I can not remember being so low at home when I could not bear to see anyone, all are welcome.

I am exercising more, eating more and concentrating more, and my meals now come on plates rather than on tiny glass dishes. I still can not eat with June as I am revolted by the smell of food but there is some improvement. The usual is happening with the steroids, constipation and I have an uncomfortable feeling that more is going in than is coming out. I have only been eating solid food for 5 days, so progress is being made.

The other great news is that Peter Reid, the Messiah of Roker Park is going to sign a contract shortly which is just the news to hear for certain patients in need of good cheer.

Tuesday 23 May

I have seen Dr Marcus and he is pleased with the way the platelets are coming up, now 29. This did not seem much to me, but he made the point that the treatment had only been going for 10 days. The drugs had to firstly correct the problem of my cannibalisation before the platelets could grow. It is a pity there is no cure for impatience.

Things do not appear to be going well and I think I am heading for a setback. I have set myself a target to be up and about by Ascot week, but already I doubt if I can get anywhere near that. I now have indigestion all the time, I was hoping it was due to the constipation but nothing seems to help and all the time the pain is getting worse.

Dr Marcus thinks it could be reaction to the steroids and the plan is to reduce them week by week over the next four weeks. It is important to keep taking the damned things to help grow the platelets but I just don't know if I will be able to hang on. The pain is getting worse all the time and is now almost constant. Antacids are useless I may as well be taking Smarties, and still the pain grinds on. I have now stopped eating so the problem can not be digestive, my bet is still those evil steroids.

Still, nobody said it would be easy.

Wednesday 24 May

I had to see Dr Weare eventually who switched the steroids. The new ones cost three times as much but do not irritate the stomach. It begs the question of course why was I given the others in the first place. Also rang Dr Marcus and he said to try and hang on for 24 hours. I think that he was thinking aloud and mentioned that it could be an ulcer. Wonderful news. He then came back to his original idea that it was gastric irritation which would go away when the original pills left my system. I suppose if it were an ulcer it is so easy to correct now that it would have been no problem.

I thought back to when my father was alive and the trouble he had with his ulcers. It is a tragic thing that it is all I remember about him, being doubled up with pain all the time. Some people seem to have all the bad luck that is going. He had a happy time until the war, but five years in the Durham Light Infantry did him no good at all. After coming out of the army he struggled on for a few years and died aged 42, never to see his children grow up, let alone grandchildren. Comparing my illness to either of my parents it is clear that I have had an easy time.

Myeloma and me

In the meantime, my pain is shattering and I can think of nothing else, I get no respite at all. The only pain I have had is back pain when I have been overdoing things in the garden and this is at least comparable. I am pleased that we never keep any sleeping pills in the house. I could see myself taking one, and then in a painful haze taking another by mistake.

Friday 26 May

Dr Marcus has said that we should stop the steroids and I am sure that I will benefit from this once they leave my system. It turned out to be the worst night of my life and ended with calling out the doctor on call, Dr Keller. I can see his point, he does not know what is my problem and does not want to treat an unknown illness. The pain I describe to him cannot be solely gastritis and he can do nothing in the meantime.

He gave me an inoculation which at least knocked me out for the night, and that was so good. In seconds the jab took effect and I felt myself gently floating away, a wonderful sensation. The trouble was, came the morning, back came the grinding pain.

Sunday 28 May

The last two days have been pain racked torment. I had to have the emergency doctor out both nights and they both agreed that the problem was not simply gastritis and could only suggest more powerful painkillers. I will now try anything and although I hate the idea of steroids, it may be vital and I may have to carry on.

At the moment it is agony to drink, move or sit still, and I am very close to despair, and simply giving up. It is a good job that giving up is not an option. I would think that there are illnesses which depend on the co-operation of the patient, but this is not one of them. The pain is so bad that there is no chance of just slipping away, there is a constant reminder.

Monday 29 May

All of the doctors who were sure that gastritis was not my sole problem were vindicated in one fell swoop. June noticed it at once when I took my shirt off, tracks of Shingles starting from my chest, under the arm and finishing round my back.

Now that the doctors knew what they were against, they whipped into action, and I had a prescription in 20 minutes, and the right treatment within 30. All mention of me going to Harlow as an emergency was forgotten, thankfully. If I have to go anywhere, I want it to be Addenbrooke's or The Evelyn, as they both know my history, but in the event it was not necessary. My G.P's have been terrific, and I had my first relief from the worst pain I have ever had and slept part of the night, much relieved and more confident.

Pain like this, unrelenting is totally exhausting, thank goodness that is over. I have had all I need of cowering on the settee, with a blanket round me, central heating on, shivering with cold and hurting.

Friday 2 June

Still going downhill. I had a fall which in retrospect could have been very nasty. We have double doors in our lounge which are glass. I got up to go to the kitchen, and keeled over, going down on my knees first, then forward hitting my head on the door frames. A foot either side, and it would have been glass, and it would have been an unusual line on a tombstone "This was supposed to be safety glass".

I am becoming dispirited and minor things assume an importance which they do not merit. My constipation is still with me but when I go to the toilet I pass a little mucous as well. I then have to clean myself up which causes my rump to be very sore, and so we go on. I find the whole thing undignified and degrading.

June has been wonderful as always. My G.P's have been great, but I have never felt so miserable. I only seem to perk up when June comes into the room, I may have to get her to walk round the house so that she is coming into the room more often.

What with the platelet problem and the steroids and the gastritis and the shingles and now the sore behind, my recovery is back about two months. I am supposed to go to Ascot at the end of the month. There is more chance of a rocking horse having a pee.

Saturday 3 June

More medical supplies have arrived, suppositories and Anusol. The Anusol was soothing, but I may as well have pushed the suppositories up my behind for all the good they did. I must be a latent comedian, I have waited years to use that.

Having achieved another first in my life, the dreaded suppositories, things have started to improve although painfully. It will be nice to be able to cure one of my problems and this is getting to be the classic example of the cure being worse than the disease.

Sunday 4 June

The torpedoes have done their work and the constipation is cured. I am performing normally, and oh, the joy of it. They say that the simple pleasures are the best and perhaps because I have had few pleasures recently, it feels good. Just so I don't regress back into my cocky stage here comes some more aggravation. I now have a pain which starts as a pain in my gums, moving up round the ears to the forehead and temple. I am starting to believe in a Divine Being. Every time he sees me improving, I get a swift kick in the groin. The churchmen say that our God is a jealous God, I think he is a sadistic bugger too.

I had two falls overnight, one of them very bad. In one of my toilet trips, I had just finished thankfully, and simply folded up from the knees. I came down on the wash basin, luckily trapping an arm underneath which protected my ribs before hitting my head and back on the bath. The commotion woke June up and we managed between us to stand me up and she tried to walk me back to bed. The same thing happened again only this time I fell against the wardrobe door which was not nearly so bad. This time I gave up trying to walk and crawled to the bed in an admittedly undignified, but safe fashion. Also, for the time being, no more standing up in the toilet, Oh the indignity. Apparently the painkillers can have this reaction, causing giddiness so I am taking no more of them. I may get less sleep, but stand a better chance of staying alive.

This reminded me of Ian's first attempt at grown up toilet habits. We were in a public toilet when I heard him shout, 'Dad look at me!' and started to turn round. A semicircle of men were soon running in all directions.

Tuesday 6 June

Returned from seeing Dr Marcus, Tuesday is Evelyn day. Simply travelling sixty miles as a passenger in a comfortable car, totally exhausts me. I told him that I felt worse than I did when leaving hospital, and he agreed that I was probably right. He always has something good to say, however, and said that my state was normal and would improve. He said that my weakness was understandable, but weakness is a relative term. When I talk of weakness, I mean having to sit down all the time in the toilet, and whilst cleaning my teeth, not being able to push a pill through the blister, the list goes on. Any one of these exertions usually means a lie down to recover.

Although Dr Marcus is up-beat and confident, which is reassuring, he makes no attempt to deny that this is a serious setback. I am back to minus square one and we are now looking towards July as a target for reasonable fitness. He thinks that stopping the steroids was a good move as we are sure that they were causing me grief but there is a sting in that particular tale. It is important to wean patients off steroids gradually but because of the effect they were having on me, on balance it was better for me to come off them "cold turkey". It is not an easy course to take but they were doing so much damage that it was unavoidable.

The plan now is to come off all tablets and to return in five weeks. In the meantime my indispensable G.P. Dr Weare will call and take blood samples each week, and organise the results to be faxed through to Dr Marcus. Apart from that I need to do whatever exercise I can, but the crux of the whole thing is to eat. This disturbs me, as far from eating more my appetite is getting less and less.

Still, Dr Marcus is confident so I do not propose to let him down by whining, and to disappoint all the people who are working hard to help me. "Nil illegitemi, non carborundum", roughly translated, "Don't let them grind you down."

Chapter Five – Down Into Despair

Wednesday 7 June

I am losing confidence, I still feel very weak and wobbly and I won't have a bath if June is not in the house. I am afraid that I could have an accident getting out on my own and could lie there for ages. My food intake is dreadful, even though I really am trying. I was almost a trencherman before and now a few cornflakes, a couple of biscuits and a one inch square of fish pie is my daily ration. The Build up or Complan make up the calories to an extent but after a while it tastes like liquid Polyfilla and is revolting. Barry was here once when I was trying to drink this gloop and the expression on his face said it all. No words were needed.

On the exercise front, this is virtually nil. I am simply trying to keep warm, with the central heating on, wrapped in a blanket, and shivering. I am starting to wonder what purpose there is in all of this. There was an American philosopher who said "Some days I sits and thinks, some days I just sits", he is like a kindred spirit at the moment. I need to be convinced what good I am doing just lying here with no improvement in sight, and the feeling that every day, I am a little weaker.

Thursday 8 June

Still no change, still as weak as a kitten and freezing cold. Managed the small scraps of biscuits with an inch square of chicken this time. I managed to shuffle round the house a little. By leaving the doors open, I can go from the lounge into the dining room, then to the kitchen, then the hall and back into the lounge making a circuit of perhaps 50 feet. I think carpet shuffling should be recognised for the feat it is. There are some really daft sports in the Olympic games now; perhaps there is room for one more.

I even managed to go up and down the stairs twice, eat your heart out Charles Atlas.

Friday 9 June

I feel that I am going downhill, and very much like I was when I got thrush. Also my throat jaw and ears hurt and the shooting pains in my temple are still there. My hope is that it is not something else brewing up, or I will be put back another few weeks.

There is a crazy logic in all of this. If I keep going back a few weeks, eventually I will be back before I was ill. Back to my carpet shuffling and trying to eat. The amount I am managing, if a mouse ate it, there would be too little to make a dropping.

Saturday 10 June

Today is Derby day and we got a 2nd and a 3rd. I seem to remember the Derby was always in the middle of the week, perhaps my brain is now going as well. I am trying to read to keep my brain active and have been noticing pains in what used to be my biceps. It could be that in my unbelievably weak state this is muscle strain from holding books up. At least now I have the energy and interest to read, so perhaps I shouldn't grumble.

I am worried that food is starting to revolt me completely and this would be serious. When I am eating tiny amounts there is always the hope that I will increase, but if it stops altogether, then I am going down. Apart from the Build ups, I am managing soup and corn flakes, not much for a growing lad.

Still trying to keep mobile I managed to walk to the bottom of the garden and back with the aid of a stick and then had a lie down. I find that going to bed during the day is vital as when I have tried to do without I simply sleep in a chair so it is better to go to bed.

Sunday 11 June

High spot of the day, Jim and Judy called. I look forward to my friends calling although it tires me, but Jim coming is a bonus as I know how much of an effort he would have had to make. Apart from this, they are really good company and it was great to see them.

The weather was vile and I had to stay indoors but I am so weak that I could not have got very far. I am trying to remember a sign of encouragement but have failed. To press a point, I suppose my exercise is slightly more, but in every other respect, I am standing still or going backwards.

Monday 12 June

Dr Weare called to take the blood sample and had time for a chat which I always find to be useful. I feel very low at times and other times close to tears and he says that this is normal. Furthermore, in his opinion, coming off the steroids as I had to is almost sure to cause a severe loss of appetite. The loss of muscle is also understandable but he is sure it would come back although it would take ages, particularly my Quads. He also said that in 15 years, I am the first myeloma patient to have survived.

This brings home how much has been achieved during one youngish doctor's career. His experience in hospitals during this time would have been without transplants and less knowledge of chemo. I am grateful to the clever people who have developed my treatment over the years, just ready for me.

Food intake is no better and I am maintaining a bit of exercise. Dr Weare tells me not to be afraid to exhaust myself. I could do that by turning the page of a book too vigorously.

Tuesday 13 June

I am sure that I am eating less and I wonder if June is losing patience. It is awful when she tries to bring me food, both of us knowing how vital it is, to find that I can not face it. I see the hurt in her eyes, and I can do nothing to help. Any subterfuge I can think of I employ. If it looks like June has forgotten my afternoon biscuit I will not remind her, the revulsion is so strong.

I am now being sick after my tiny scraps of food, things are not going well.

Wednesday 14 June

There is now a constant pain which is the aftermath of the shingles. I would like to meet the person who invents all these illnesses. For the first time, which is incredible, June dropped her guard and niggled at me this morning. That made me depressed all day. I have found that I have lost mental strength as well as physical, and setbacks are very hard to take. June has been truly magnificent throughout, a five foot mountain and the thought that I had upset her was almost too much to take. She no doubt shrugged it off in minutes, but it left a dark cloud over me for hours.

I depend on her totally and how quickly I get over this thing will be due mostly to her. I owe her everything.

Thursday 22 June

I have decided to write up my notes weekly as not much happens day by day. It is June's birthday on the 23rd, on Royal Ascot day. A group of friends have combined and we save up during the year by standing order, and use the money to go to Ascot. The money pays for the transport, champagne lunch, overnight stay in a Hotel with Dinner on the way back and whatever is left is given back for betting money. It is a great day out even for people like me, who are not particularly keen on horse racing, but sadly not this year. Ascot is like a Cup Final at Wembley, Wimbledon, the Olympic Games, the enjoyment is down to the occasion as much as the event. In fact to be harsh, some of these sports are now total boredom, and it is only the sense of occasion which makes them worthwhile.

My shingles pain is unrelenting, and the thrush makes my mouth slimy. No wonder I am finding eating such a struggle. The platelets are coming up nicely, and Dr Weare and Dr Marcus are to get their heads together to see if they can alter the treatment at all.

Thursday 29 June

I am following the usual routine, blood samples, then my doctors discuss the result and we go forward from there. The platelets are now 29 and if they had been at this level 6 weeks ago I would not have needed the damned steroids. Dr Marcus now thinks that we should stop all drugs and let the chemo flush itself away. The signs are there, beard growth etc. and I will never argue with anyone telling me to stop taking pills.

At last I am improving, albeit very slowly. One day I went for a walk twice, a magnificent feat. My improvements may be laughable to a fit person, but are very real to me. Going up to bed is very tiring, and I have had to flop on the bed for a few minutes before getting up to close the curtains. One night, without realising I had done it, I walked over to close the curtains without stopping.

Small though it may be, it is a concrete sign that things are getting ever so slightly better, and after weeks of getting worse day by day, I am proud of myself. I feel that another come-back is on the way, I will soon have more than Frank Sinatra.

Thursday 6 July

Platelets are now 39, to the delight of all concerned, and I can now look forward to seeing Dr Marcus to discuss what progress we have made. We are far from the beer and skittles stage but I go out every day for a walk come what may. I am still eating virtually nothing. The food I am eating tastes of wildly different things. I had a strawberry and it tasted like petrol.

The shingles, like the pain is always with me, I sleep badly, and now small brown spots are appearing all over my legs and arms. Dr Weare thinks it could be Psoriasis, but he is not sure and as it is not life threatening, we will ignore it. It doesn't bother me, if I am going to work my way through the medical dictionary, let's be having you, I will take you all on.

Tuesday 11 July

Saw Dr Marcus again and he is pleased with the way things are going. My hair is growing and my finger nails are growing now and pushing the dead nails out. The chemo killed off the nail beds and this is a sure sign that my body is starting to repair itself. He thinks that I could be one month away from normality and were it not for the shingles he thinks I could have been back to work. For my part I don't agree at all, but am pleased to go along with the principle that I am on the mend.

I really think that the food intake is the crux to everything, and far from improving I am getting worse. The regular appointments don't bother me particularly apart from the bone marrow aspirations. Dr Marcus tends to re-assure me and Linda cheers me up so I am happy to go but the journeys are becoming a nightmare. I have no flesh, not a trace of fat or muscle and I am literally sitting on bone. Every movement of the car hurts me.

Still, things are not going badly. My weight is just about holding, the shingles is still bad, but no thrush, no visits planned for six weeks, no drugs, no blood tests, no blood marrow aspirations planned, life is good.

Saturday 22 July

It is my 56th birthday on the 23rd, I may ask for a Complan cake. What a calamitous year this has been but at least things are heading my way now. The weather has turned and it is a lovely summer day. Alf and Eileen called en route to Redhill and we even sat in the garden for a while which was very pleasant. I still sleep badly, the shingles still hurt and my weight is drifting away, now 9st 8lbs, which is the weight I was when I was married in 1963. I am only 5ft 8, but I was built like a pipe cleaner although I was as fit as a butcher's dog.

I look far worse now as I head for Biafran proportions, but I want to eat like a human not fill my calorie deficit up with Complan or Build up. There is also a substance which will mix with food and is undetectable but virtually doubles the calories. I will be amazed if I am not being fed this stuff surreptitiously but it seems to be having little effect.

Dr Marcus thinks that my appetite should show signs in about another month. Let us hope that he is right.

Friday 28 July

Now suffering from boredom, nothing is happening. I am still keeping up the exercise but still not sleeping, and still not eating. The weight is still drifting downwards, now 9st 4, which I don't mind too much as it seems to be a controlled loss rather than a crash. My mystery rash is still there and three doctors have now seen it but are not concerned in any way. Each in their own way have said we should take no further action on it but I am less polite. If it is not hurting, itching or spreading, bugger it.

I am now reduced to taking a pillow with me when I ride in the car or sit on the settee to try and keep a layer between me and the bone.

Monday 31 July

Slightly weaker, which could be the combination of no sleep, and no food. A few weeks ago, I just could not keep warm no matter how I tried. Now I am over this and the weather is glorious and of course I am now too hot. I have just realised that my saliva glands are not working which is making it very difficult to swallow and I think that I am now starting to lose the swallowing reflex. Never mind, if I learned to gargle I am sure I can re-learn to swallow when the time comes. I have been trying odd snacks and anything salty like crisps nearly blow my head off, the salt taste is so exaggerated.

My finger nails are now very strong, the nasal hair has returned stronger than before and my hair has returned exactly the same colour as before and the same style, if my hair can be dignified by describing it as such. It is a lot finer now and is almost like silk. One of these days, I suppose I will have to get it cut, but at least I am lucky there, as a friend does it for me. I would find it hard to go to one of those Unisex places, it is just not my style at all. What became of the old fashioned men's barbers? Pure nostalgia, the fly blown mirror above a cracked basin, the chair with the stuffing coming out of the arms, the lino worn away with countless shuffling feet and the varnish worn away from the drawer in which the "packets of three" are kept. The modern places lack that indefinable touch of squalor essential to a barber's shop.

Wednesday 9 August

I disappointed myself and went to the surgery for pain killers for the shingles. This was very much against the grain but I cannot sleep, or even sit for long. I felt I had to do something. At least Dr Keller came up with a name for my mystery rash, he thinks it could be Psoriasis, the same as Dr Weare. At least I can put away ludicrous thoughts. It did cross my mind that as I seem to be working my way through the medical dictionary, that melanoma is close to myeloma.

It is our Wedding Anniversary shortly and the celebration this year will be subdued. I regard this as a true celebration rather than a birthday which is pure chance. The wedding anniversary is a celebration of something we have done deliberately. I have said many times over the years that marrying June has been the best thing I have done in my life so far. It is a shame that this year the best I can hope for is a double helping of Complan!

Tuesday 15 August

It looks like I may be heading for another setback. The strange rash is clearing, and the shingles pain appears to be moderating, although the drugs may have to be stepped up. What worried me was when I went for my normal walk. I have varied walks trying to incorporate hills, and have been quite pleased with myself. On this occasion, I had only gone 25 yards when I began to stagger and was lucky to make it back home unaided. Chris was there at the time and I don't think she realised that I had been out and had come back. I didn't feel particularly hot but my temperature was showing 38.7, and there was nothing for it but to go back to the Evelyn. Dr Marcus is not too concerned about the infection, and is now wondering if my eating problem is due to a liver infection.

I think that I am being lazy and not repairing as fast as others and it is annoying if I have picked up something else. Dr Marcus follows his usual style, and says that if it does turn out to be liver damage, it can be cured. I don't doubt him, but I am shying away from a liver biopsy. Probably 90% of words are quite innocuous, but put biopsy on the end and they assume a malevolence in my eyes.

From the beginning of this illness I have resolved to be as good a patient as I can; I am sure it helps recovery and makes it easier all round. Now, however, I am losing my confidence and starting to feel very low, being called back into hospital and problems possibly looming. The most ironic thing is that the Evelyn is known for the standard of the food and of course I am still not eating.

Wednesday 16 August

Dr Weare called round, and advised me to stop taking the drugs for the shingles pain for a completely sensible reason. If they are testing the liver for damage, it is self defeating to have the residue of drugs in there, so no pain killers. He also said that liver and lung problems are common complications and that I should not worry.

Dr Marcus has arranged for a cat scan on Thursday, which should help find out what is going on. The worst part of the cat scan was drinking the fluid beforehand and waiting for it to get into my system. The scanning process is quite interesting, totally painless, just a little awkward trying to keep still all the time. It is probable that I have a lung infection which is pushing my temperature to 39°, and a liver infection which may be the cause of the anorexia which is a posh way of saying not eating. After the cat scan I have to stay overnight at the Evelyn with another stay later on.

I am feeling very low, depressed and pessimistic. It seems that as soon as I even begin to make headway along comes something else to take me down. If things follow the usual course I will bounce back very soon but I really do feel very low and dejected. For the first time I am beginning to wonder what will happen if the lung and liver infections can't be cured: "where does that leave me then ?"

I am too tired to look for it but a copy of my will is somewhere in the house. On a similar black-humoured vein, I am very fond of *Adagio* by Tomaso Albinoni, and said in jest to Andie many years ago that I wanted it played at my funeral. I still like the piece but for some reason I don't play it any more.

Friday 18 August

The cat scan was fascinating and the results were semi-acceptable. It showed that I do not have a liver infection which is a great relief except that we still don't know what is stopping me eating. The other news is that I have pneumonia, which was not so bad as June had warned me that it was what they were looking for and that the cure was standard. Of course Lucky Jim asserted himself, as there is only one strain of the illness which necessitates hospital care and my fungal pneumonia was the one.

I am therefore back in the Evelyn for ten days, possibly longer. It is bad timing, as the Sister on the ward where June works is seriously ill and will be off for months. The hospital will not replace her so June has to organise all of that as well as worrying about me. Still, nobody said it would be easy.

Saturday 19 August

Dr Marcus called to see me early, but had little to add to the information of last night. The total treatment will take between four and six weeks, but it is possible that after ten days I may be able to go home and continue it there. As I am a long term patient, I have been given a much better room overlooking the garden which is very pleasant.

I had a cannula fitted into a vein and although I was dreading it, I hardly noticed it going in and treatment began in earnest. My diet now is liquid but I had mushroom soup which tasted very much like mushroom. This could be the sign I have been waiting for. It might be imagination but I feel a little better, always the eternal optimist; still, if you are a Sunderland supporter, that is a prerequisite.

What is not imagination, however, is the return of the diarrhoea, so now I collect it in a small bucket for testing. It is not as bad as before, in that I now have control and can get into the toilet. The whole procedure is an unwanted addition to my problems and I find it degrading. Luckily, I am the only one who thinks that.

Sunday 20 August

Porridge for breakfast which I did not enjoy as it seemed to be made with water, but the taste was correct. I now want to take advantage of the food, increase my exercise and, it can't just be wishful thinking, I do feel better. The cannula then decided to break down, and I ended up having one in my right hand which is slightly more awkward as I am right handed, but what the hell.

Tomorrow I want to start another comeback, unless fate has anything else in store for me.

Myeloma and me

Monday 21 August

Slept quite well, it was a much better night. Dr Marcus called on his early morning round and he is quite pleased. He also called in the afternoon when June was there which is always a good thing. June understands the intricacies of the treatment far better than I and it is better when they can talk to each other. The diarrhoea is still a bit of a problem but the temperature is now normal so things are doing well.

This strain of pneumonia apparently is dangerous if not tackled promptly. The treatment contains potassium and if the drip runs low it could cause kidney damage which I can well do without. Dr Marcus is still keen on me going home with a pump and I am all for that but it will mean that I will have to have a new line in on Thursday. My memories of the last line are still quite vivid so I was relieved to learn from the nurses that it would be inserted under sedation.

Tuesday 22 August

Temperature is stable, diarrhoea almost gone, but we had trouble with the pump all day. If the mix is not right, it is dangerous and the pump has to be watched during the day. After the first one stopped it was replaced, and this one was just the same. It looked like pilot error to me, but we left it on gravity feed all day, and that gave no problems at all.

I had a walk round the hospital, ate a little food, and the only niggle was the heat. It is ironic that for so long I have struggled to keep warm, it is now glorious weather and I can not stand the heat. Whether heat irritates the shingles or not I don't know, but I have been in torment with it all day, it is about time it departed.

Wednesday 23 August

I was trundled off to x-ray, and the infection is better. Nothing to stop having my line put in, and the surgeon called to see me. It will be a Hickman line, which is the third variety I have had, and he is quite blasé about the whole thing. He will simply go in through the neck and come out further down. A doddle.

Like a clown I forgot to tell him that the shingles is active on the right side, and to ask him to operate on the left. One of the sisters said that she would let him know. I hope she remembers otherwise it will be painful later on.

A strange thing: I am still frightened of needles even after my many years of blood donation and all the procedures here and at Addenbrooke's, but I was calm and relaxed about tomorrow. I know that the procedure is very minor but it is the first time I have ever been in a theatre. Never mind, I feel fine about it.

Thursday 24 August

My confidence about the operation was correct, I was given a sedative in my room and the next thing I remember is being on the trolley on the way back. I spent the rest of the day drifting in and out of sleep which is usual after a general. There is a slight pain at the site of the incision which is on the left side away from my shingles. The only problem is my voice which has almost gone. This is a nuisance.

When Dr Marcus called it made me more monosyllabic than normal, but he is still talking about me going home on Saturday. A strange thing which may have been imagination was that he asked me a few times if I had anything to tell him, but he asked in a way that made me think he was expecting me to . It was odd but could just as easily have been reaction from the anaesthetic and nonsense on my part.

Chapter Six – Heavy Breathing

Friday 25 August

My throat is no better and both the surgeon and his anaesthetist called to see me. The normal procedure was followed which involves holding back the vocal cords for a while, and the loss of voice sometimes happens. The nerve is damaged and takes a while to recover. My obvious question was how long is a while but there is no definite time span. It had better hurry up while I still have some reputation left. I tried to telephone Dow Stoker where I work, and they thought I was a heavy breather.

The Hickman line has three ports, of which only one is needed. It did occur to me that a simple central line with only one port would have done and saved me all this bother. The answer, of course, is that this line is more durable, wider, and gives less trouble but things like this are starting to make me nervous. I am starting to wonder when these problems are going to stop and let me get back to fitness. I am now such a long way off my best that I wonder if I will be ever completely over it.

I am just as convinced that I will make a full recovery from the myeloma, but the chemo has hammered me so much with the unrelated problems that keep cropping up, that I wonder if I will get back to being the man I was before. There surely must be a time when the damage to the system is so much that only a reduced level of recovery is possible. My system has certainly taken a hammering, and I am so far off full fitness, it seems to be an awfully long uphill road ahead of me.

Dr Marcus called with some good and bad news. Firstly, he sees no reason why I should not go home tomorrow but if the throat is no better someone will look down with a mirror. This fills me with dread, and I hope to hell I do get better. If there was any better incentive I would like to know what it is. I speak in a sort of a sultry whisper and although I can just about make myself understood it is hard work and I am virtually shouting all the time.

Saturday 26 August

It was an awful journey, but I got home safely. The "home-made" drip works perfectly so we should be fine from now on in our tiny cottage hospital. I need something to shake me out of the mood of despondency I am in. Gradually, almost without realising it, I have let myself slide. To be sure, things are not going well, but up to now I have always put on a front: it is becoming difficult now.

My voice is still no better and we have three doctors at the Evelyn who are not sure what it is and when it will recover, and this demonstrates the way I am now. Previously I would have been impatient but would have been asking when it would be better. Now in unguarded moments I am accepting that it will be permanent and that more complications are lined up ready. I need to snap out of this, and I will, but I feel that I have been clouted over the head so much it is difficult to see the way out.

Sunday 27 August

One of my shortest and most waspish notes. Voice no better, appetite declining, now 8st 13, and growing weaker. June has to help me out of the bath, becoming dizzy and breathless.

Monday 28 August

All of the above, the same or worse, we will have to see what Dr Marcus says on Tuesday.

Ian borrowed our car yesterday and wrapped it up. It is not too badly damaged, and Ian was not hurt but it is one more thing for June to deal with. I have always handled such things in the past and it is good to see Ian helping with this and other "male" tasks.

The football season has slunk up almost unheralded, I must be worse than I thought. I failed to see a single game at Roker

Park last season, and apart from being abroad in the R.A.F. this is the first season I have missed since I started to go at the age of nine. By common consent we are doing pretty well for a team which was almost relegated last year.

We are through one round of a Mickey Mouse cup which started off as the League Cup and has had many names since then, all dafter than the previous. There already is a proper cup, the F.A. Cup, which is the best cup competition in the world, so why did the F.A. not make the new cup mean something, like a Great Britain cup. Let us have the Scots, Irish and Welsh clubs in and give it some interest. In case I should be accused of sour grapes, as we normally do badly, I was saying just the same when we were in the final against Norwich and lost of course. I think the F.A. has the most appropriate initials possible.

Tuesday 29 August

I had another x-ray which showed the infection still clearing up. Dr Marcus does not suspect liver damage but I have to see a specialist later on in the week to give a further opinion. It seems that the tablets I am taking to ensure that the liver keeps flushed out are causing some mischief, so we have stopped the diuretics which should bring a great improvement.

I still have to ensure that my bladder works overtime, so I am drinking copious amounts of fluid. During my nocturnal trips, of which there are many, I am feeling giddy and have almost fallen a few times. At least I have managed to stay upright and manage on my own.

Wednesday 30 August

Dr Marcus is pleased with the blood tests, so I may not have to be admitted. I still have to see Dr Jameson later on in the week but I will not be going to the theatre so I feel that I am getting off lightly.

Thursday 31 August

Dr Marcus telephoned to tell me to stop taking the current treatment as it is apparently causing an electrolyte imbalance, and is the probable reason for me feeling so rotten. I am a classic example of the cure being worse than the disease. It is incredible when I remember that I have never had any symptom of the illness, perhaps it is just as well.

I will now be admitted on Friday, and there is a new treatment for me which is horribly expensive but is supposed to be excellent and has few side effects. What a pity I was not given this in the first place.

Friday 1 September

Saw Dr Jameson, and he said that although my throat problem should not have happened, it was no one's fault and was simply something which happens from time to time. If that is the case they should arrange to share these things out, I have had my share. All of the correct procedures were followed in the theatre, nothing went wrong, it was just one of those things. I wondered afterwards if Dr Jameson wanted to see me to judge my reaction to it all, but the subject was never raised.

He managed to get an appointment for me to see Mr Ellis, the E.N.T. specialist, the man with the dreaded mirror. Although it was ghastly it was better than I had dreaded and the news was not bad. He said that one vocal cord nerve was damaged but that it would heal itself. If I wanted to there was an operation he could do which would cure the problem but advised me to wait.

Paul is coming home from Australia in two days after being there for six months, and I am getting myself upset because I won't be able to talk to him properly. I was thinking nonsense, like I had failed him as a father; it was bad enough not being able to meet him, but now this. Thank goodness there was nobody to confide this to, they would be looking for a rubber room.

I do find though that I am not in any way robust, not physically or mentally. Any small thing, like Paul's homecoming, and not being able to speak properly assumes gigantic proportions when in truth it is simply not important at all, simply a minor inconvenience.

Saturday 2 September

Dr Marcus is growing more cautious and I think he wants me to stay in for the whole treatment. If that is what is required, so be it. We are all on the same side in this. It is apparently a problem in mixing the new mixture and only a pharmacist is supposed to do it. I am sure June could do it, my little wife can do anything, but it is more a case of whether she will be allowed to. Anyway, watch this space.

I saw my latest x-ray today, and although Dr Marcus is happy with it, to me my right lung looks awful. Stick with the experts, this is no place for uninformed amateurs.

Sunday 3 September

Dr Marcus has threatened me with an exploratory tube into my lungs if things do not improve, so I got better immediately. Words like biopsy, throat mirror and exploratory tube seem to do wonders for my recovery. Seriously, I am feeling slightly better in walking and breathing; the improvement is very slight but it is there.

Dr Marcus wants me to stay a few more days just to make sure. If I do deteriorate, or something new crops up, he doesn't want me an hour's drive away and be half dead when I get here. I will concede that point.

Paul came to see me today and he looks and sounds terrific. We managed to converse in a fashion and he has up to date news of Andie and Steve who are doing very well. I get tired talking and must make sure I get plenty of sleep to try and keep my strength up.

Monday 4 September

I saw the physio today, and the exercises shattered me, which must be a good thing in the end. My legs have always been strong, and even now when they look like spaghetti I can still walk. What is strange though is that when I look down I get laboured breathing and giddiness. I must keep the exercises going even though it is hard. What is not helping is my almost total lack of appetite. This worries me, I even feel ashamed and yet I can do nothing to help. I fully understand the tricks that anorexics get up to but our situations are entirely different in that I would love to eat but can't.

I have said that June should give special attention to Paul for a while. It is going to be difficult coming back from Australia to finish his last year at university, and he needs her to help him out. Of course this means that she spends less time with me and I miss her badly but it is the right thing to do.

Dr Marcus is still pleased with the way things are going generally, so I am regaining my confidence. One strange thing happened which I am still not completely sure about. I know when the drip needs to be changed and there is a set way of doing it. Without my trying to remember it I have become aware of the procedure and it has become almost a rhythmic pattern. This day it was completely different and I realised that I had never seen the nurse before and she did the drip in a totally different way and took less than half the time to do it. She may have cut corners which may bring increased chances of infection but my recollection is hazy. Of course it could have been a saboteur from P.P.P. trying to cut the bill down.

Our friends son and his wife have their first child today and I remembered a piece of doggerel from my grandmother. It is odd how daft thoughts get into one's head at unguarded moments. She always maintained that as one person joins the human race another leaves it. Thanks Gran, nice one.

Myeloma and me

Tuesday 5 September

Very slight improvement, but after the exercises, every apology for a muscle is sore. My physio is insisting that she accompanies me on my walks, so clearly she is keeping a close eye on me. Everything seems to be running all right and Dr Marcus is still looking at ways of letting me go home. He now thinks I am on the road to recovery. In the past this has been the harbinger of doom.

I have four visitors coming in tomorrow and although I can't speak properly and it tires me, it is just so good to have them. It may be that visitors give a sense of normality. I certainly enjoy the conversation and it means so much. Non patients cannot really grasp the significance of visitors, they really are helpful.

Today, I ate a tiny piece of meat, twice. I feel like Henry VIII.

Wednesday 6 September

My exercises carry on, some on the bed (we used to call this Egyptian P.T. in the forces), and the usual walks round the corridors. I only get breathless when I go too fast or when I talk, so I am reasonably pleased, but it is the stairs tomorrow. This is the North Face of the Eiger and must be mastered before I go home. I am confident of doing this but I am not too sure about going home. Conflicting emotions are in force. I really want to go home but my confidence has taken a dip and I am starting to wonder if an extra day or two might do me good.

Black humour abounds. The rope for the blind had twisted itself in the wind into the shape of a noose. This swung backwards and forwards all day creating surreal images. Also, someone died today and the atmosphere has physically changed, a pall is hanging over the ward and yet nothing has been spoken to cause this. Tales of the supernatural.

Thursday 7 September

Went to the Eiger with my Physio and went at a snail's pace, 3/4 of the way up the stairs. I felt that I could have gone to the top, but noticed the loose bannister rail at the top. This is probably due to people dragging themselves up by hand. Maggie says that she was surprised that I have done so well judging by my emaciated appearance so that makes me feel better.

I have been giving more thought to going home and whether I have become a wimp or semi-institutionalised I know not but I would feel happier for a few extra days here. Significantly, June feels the same. Dr Marcus was still willing to let me go, but when we told him our decision he seemed to look relieved and pleased. It may have been the right decision.

Friday 8 September

Still gaining strength very slowly and becoming bored and impatient. Dr Marcus told me that my kidney function had returned to normal which was great apart form the fact that I had no recollection of being told that it wasn't. I tried a piece of fillet steak in my gastronomic quest and had got half way through when it jammed in my throat. This made me choke, then vomit, and that was the end of that fiasco, all my fault.

I am not sleeping well, not eating at all, but I don't feel as tired, let us see what I am like in a few days.

Saturday 9 September

I have always thought that men are not very bright, including this one. Having started to feel a bit stronger, I went at the exercise like a bull at a gate, strained my groin and had to go back to bed. At least I renewed my acquaintance with a young doctor from Addenbrooke's who was surprised that I had had such a rough time, but confirmed that the strain was minor.

We agreed to write this day off and start again tomorrow.

Sunday 10 September

I took things easy, just had two walks round the corridors, and up the stairs. If Dr Marcus is still happy I will go home on Tuesday and start another comeback. The trouble is that I start from a lower point each time. I am now unbelievably weak, no appetite, no libido, no energy, just totally useless. I doubt if I could look after myself now I am totally dependent on others.

The hospital has decided that June will be allowed to mix the drugs and therefore I will be able to go home sooner. She is to handle the drip when we get home and, naturally, she is keen to learn the proper way to do the sterilisation procedures, and is busy picking the brains of the nurses. June is completely confident that she can mix the drugs and can handle the drip on gravity feed so there is no problem.

Monday 11 September

Went on a long walk with the physio and felt fine apart from tiring myself trying to speak. I am a chatterer, and this enforced trappist monk existence does not go down too well. The x-rays taken this morning are fine, as was the blood test, and when I see Dr Marcus tomorrow I should go straight home afterwards.

Barry called to visit but June was late after having to deal with more problems at work. It was sad news, as it seems that her Ward Sister has died, and although she was very ill, it has a terrible effect on morale. Sue was apparently offered early retirement on the grounds of ill health but never got round to signing the forms. This was a shame as it could have made her last days a little easier. It must be hard for a nurse or doctor to have a very serious illness as they will be aware of all the ramifications all the time. A very sad end.

Tuesday 12 September

I returned home after a terrible journey. The courtesy car lent to us by my insurance company was very welcome but not as comfortable as our Rover. On reaching home I sank into bed and felt much better for it. June handles the drip with consummate ease so we have no problems on that score. We have the drip and all the paraphernalia in our bedroom and I can watch T.V., or read, or even attempt to eat while it is going on.

I will stop making daily notes as I am not anticipating much to happen at home, just slow steady progress.

13-16 September

The blood tests are still all right so the procedure is as before. Walk about the house, climb the stairs starting off at twice without stopping, twice a day, gradually increasing. I think I am becoming a little stronger but the food side is worrying me, I was almost in tears when I was unable to finish a tiny piece of potato. What concerns me is that I am so weak that I will be unable to fend off any bugs that are around. I am also getting emotional, not like me at all. Nobody has caught me at it yet but I suppose it will come.

One thing which is better than expected is the performance of Sunderland A.F.C. They almost went out last season but now they are doing well and are ninth in the table. We have never been as high as that for years, I just hope the players don't get nose bleeds.

17 -20 September

Still tramping up and down stairs and feel a little better, but oh so slow. I saw Dr Marcus on the 19th and he says things are fine, and that the voice "should get better", but might take three months. He also said that it was nothing to do with him, which is quite correct but I seemed to detect a note of relief when he said it. Also I wasn't too keen on the "should", but no doubt I am reading into it something which wasn't there, but I am frustrated at the lack of progress.

We have a further week of treatment at home which should put the chest right, then start investigating the lack of appetite. Officially, I am suffering from anorexia, but not nervosa, like these silly Royal lasses, but an unwanted bloody annoying strength sapping nuisance. In the meantime I continue to plod up and down stairs and I may even get outside if the weather is good enough.

21 – 24 September

I have managed to increase my stair climbing to four times per day, four times without stopping. It makes me out of breath, but I recover quickly so I am quite pleased with myself. June took Paul back to university at Hull and I was worried every minute she was away. She is at least as good a driver as I used to be, but I still worried. Barry and Judy both called while she was away, keeping a thinly disguised "eye", and it was, as always, good to see them.

My mouth has started to fill up with phlegm which is not bad if I can spit it out, but if I swallow it I am sick, I hate these undignified episodes, but it could be the pneumonia coming away. June lost her temper for only the second time. When the drip was going in she brought a meal upstairs. The smell made me retch and by the time I had set off to be sick, she had slammed the door and stormed off.

I was deeply ashamed and detest upsetting her, I can see the anguish in her eyes at every mealtime, it really is almost unbearable. On this occasion I ended up sobbing. It must be terrible for her to see me wasting away. The Complan provides almost all of my calorie intake, but I am now down to 8st 6.

Incidentally, if you only have one vocal cord working it is impossible to cry properly. I am becoming a mine of useless information.

25 – 27 September

Still climbing stairs and I feel better even though the recovery is almost imperceptible. I have been back to the Evelyn, and the x-rays are better, and Dr Marcus is pleased with my slow but steady progress. He is, however, becoming worried about my eating. What a slowcoach, I have been worried for months.

The plan now is to wait until the drugs are finished (three days) to see if that is the cause. If not we will have to consider a liver biopsy. See what I mean, we get one thing sorted out, only for something else to come along and I am getting weaker all the time. I have arranged to go back in a month, but if things are not going well, in two weeks.

Thursday 28 September

I saw Dr Marcus and appreciated his candour. I would hate a specialist who was mealy mouthed and who tried to wrap up bad news in a sycophantic way. Dr Marcus is not afraid to call a spade a shovel if he has to, and apparently, if my pneumonia had not responded to the second lot of drugs, I would have been in a lot of trouble. I did respond and it did not become life threatening but it must have been awful for June who would have known this. If a little knowledge is a dangerous thing, then quite a bit of knowledge is horrendous.

If I end up having a liver biopsy then so be it as the anticipation will be worse than the event. My G.P. tells me not to worry as it is very minor. He has given about 200 biopsies, it takes about a minute and is painless. We shall see.

29 September – 4 October

Still improving very slowly and the appetite is altering. I can eat no more, but can tolerate food that revolted me a few weeks ago. Against that I am heartily sick of the things I have been eating, so the end effect is the same.

I have taken on a little consultancy work and although at first I felt that my brain had atrophied I have struggled on. To be honest I was not satisfied with the final result but it was the best I could do in the circumstances.

I stay awake all day now and feel that I am better than I was but we will have to make a decision soon whether or not to cancel the intermediate appointment. The shingles pain is worse, the appetite is no better, we will have to decide soon.

Peter Reid must be performing miracles at Roker Park. With virtually the same squad as last season, we are winning, playing good football, and are now 6th in the League.

5 – 11 October

Very little is happening but I am keeping up with the exercise, now two walks each day plus the stairs four by four. Considering the amount of exercise I am doing it is no surprise that my weight is going down. Yesterday, I had cereal, a pot of dessert and two Build ups. I have therefore taken the decision to keep the appointment with Dr Marcus. This is the interim appointment we have made. The ground rules are that if I was significantly better I could cancel it but I can not pretend that I am better at all so needs must.

The drip is finished, and we have to find out why the liver function test is abnormal and hopefully by putting this right, it will put the appetite right. Dr Marcus rates the chances as good but we are running out of options. If this fails to work, what is the next step? The added bonus may be that if my line is taken out this may help the voice. The next step is to see the liver specialist, Dr Gimson, and although I am not looking forward to it one little bit it needs sorting out.

October 12 – 16

My exercise regime is proceeding and I feel that I am almost ready for going down to the village again. The shingles pain is bothering me and when I saw Dr Weare he offered me painkillers if I really wanted them but I am determined to take nothing which might aggravate my liver. He tells me that I also have conjunctivitis. I couldn't care less, bring them all on. In the scale of what I have been through this is not even a minor setback.

Something strange is happening, my weight is actually going up, and is now 8st 8. It could be that my metabolism is becoming used to the situation, or I could be putting on muscle from the walking. Maybe Dr Gimson will have an opinion. It turns out he is a friend of Dr Weare, and I should be able to get good treatment under the old pals act.

October 17 – 20

The only notable event is that I have achieved another milestone and have walked down to the village. I went very slowly and carefully but I got there and back with no problem. No contact from Dr Gimson.

My lads at Roker Park are doing their level best to keep my spirits up. We have just drawn with Watford and are now 4th.

October 21 – 23

I have now made the appointment to see Dr Gimson but full of trepidation at the prospect of a liver biopsy. Dr Weare tells me it is a doddle compared to the bone marrow aspiration I just hope he is right.

My exercise combined with very little food has sent my weight crashing. I am just an untidy parcel of bones, save my legs, which are not too bad. I am not going to quote my weight as 7 st something, but it is a few pounds under 8 stone.

At this weight I obviously have no fat but I am also noticeably losing muscle. This will be the hardest to correct and if it is allowed to go on for very long, the most dangerous. My lowest weight up to now is 7 stone 5, and once, I was alone in the room when the telephone rang. I was able to reach it, but could not lift it off the cradle. My obvious worry was that I was close to my involuntary muscles giving up. I resolved that I had to keep exercising and try to prevent this from happening.

October 24 – 25

I am walking greater distances now. The legs and the lungs are fine, but a dry mouth leaves me with a sickly feeling, which is not at all pleasant. My appointment with Dr Gimson was better than I had feared but we reached no firm conclusion. He is an affable, nice man, possibly more laid back than Dr Marcus, but seems just as thorough. He thinks the problem could be:

1) the residue of the drugs from the chemo sessions upsetting me, or

2) the same bug that gave me pneumonia has also caused the liver problem.

He will give me a gastroscopy next week which does not bother me too much, as I will be under sedation, and this may provide the answer. Only if that fails will he resort to a biopsy, so that must be a bonus. The degree of liver abnormality did not bother him unduly although it will still need correcting. If I am honest I was slightly disappointed not to have a firm answer today but things simply do not work that way and I should have known that. Nevertheless, we are back on another treadmill, I am hoping it is the last.

Chapter Seven – The Year Peters Out

26 October – 1 November

The months roll on, it is now November, incredible. Time passes quickly when you are enjoying yourself. Shingles is like 100 wasps, not nice at all. I saw Dr Gimson and he performed what he called an endoscopy, and it went like a charm but I was surprised how giddy and weak I was afterwards. I can not remember a single thing after getting out of the theatre but June tells me I held a conversation with Dr Gimson, answered questions and behaved normally. Obviously I perform better on drugs.

The good tidings are that with the operation I was not allowed to eat and this gave me an excuse to forego the torment of trying to force food down. There are white spots in my stomach and it seems that the stomach lining has not grown back after the ravages of the chemo. When I was at Addenbrooke's, the skin on my fingers split and eventually fell off, and was quite unpleasant. The doctors also said that the same thing would be happening to my gullet and gut so it is hardly surprising that my insides are a shambles. Knowing this has not advanced the cure for the appetite but has eliminated the liver as the cause so that again is a bonus better news than I had thought.

November 2 – 6

I am having trouble with the D.H.S.S. over my sick pay. The first reply was quite curt simply telling me that I was not entitled to Incapacity Benefit. The next stage was yet another form to be filled in, this time for Severe Disablement Benefit, wanting the same information.

Do these people not realise that they are dealing with seriously ill, vulnerable people for whom filling forms in is a torment? One question was why I had taken so long to fill the form in, when I had only had it for two days. My reply was that I was ill, ask a silly question!! They accepted it without question, proving to me that it is just a paper exercise. God help the rain forests.

On a wider front, I can never see the reason for the myriad government departments all administering their own rules and all giving separate payments out. You may be unemployed and receive one, if you are sick you receive another, and if you need help after this, there is another body. My feeling is that the government should make just one payment and dispense with all the separate offices and benefits. The horrible thing is that many of the people they are messing about are in the process of dying; what a way to go.

November 7 – 19

Nothing much is happening, at least not very quickly. I am keeping up with the walking but can do nothing with the arms and upper body. My legs are not at all bad but the shoulders and arms are just spindles. The shingles pain is still so bad that I can not use the rowing machine which would do the trick.

I am in constant pain and at times I admit it gets me down, but at times like this, I think of my mother. She was ill from the age of 14, and never had a day without pain and anxiety from then on. The only pleasure she had was the achievements of her family, passing examinations or creating grandchildren and the like. Not long before she died, she was tested to see if she was suitable for heart valve replacement which was then in its infancy. If she could have had the operation she would have been in decent health for the first time in her life but they decided she was not fit enough.

It must have been shattering for the prospect to be dangled, and then snatched away. I could see the hospital's point. They were pioneering a new procedure the last thing they wanted was early deaths. I doubt if I would have the strength of purpose to carry on, but she lasted a few more years. Her life consisted of pain, bringing up four children in poverty, nursing a war-damaged husband until he died at 42, and managing to see all of her grandchildren born. I may have had a rough time but nothing even approaching my mother's problems.

I still worry about my food intake and try as I might, nothing happens. Each meal time I try some proper food but it is a complete ordeal. Luckily, I have never had a problem eating the same meal often, but there is a limit to the number of times I can eat caramel, or soup, or ground rice.

We have made a mistake with Andie I am afraid. When my vocal cords were damaged we decided not to tell her as there was no point in worrying her unduly. One day I was in the house on my own and answered the "Australia calling" telephone, and of course she found out. She asked the perfectly reasonable question. "Why did nobody tell me?" the inference being what else was she in the dark about.

I managed to convince her that things were going well and I just hope that I am fully fit when she comes home next year. The chances must be fair. I have been through the medical dictionary once, there is nothing left to have.

November 20 – 23

News at last from Dr Gimson. I have an infection in my stomach which requires no treatment, and like the liver inflammation will correct itself. What great news, here we go again on the comeback trail. Dr Gimson said that he could fully understand why I have had problems eating but also says that when the present inflammations are cured there is no physical reason why I should not be able to eat. One problem I can see is if I am still unable to eat then and it is not a physical problem then we really are in a mess. I suppose I would have preferred it if he had found something and was able to put it right but this is the best news I have had for ages.

I see Dr Marcus on the 5th of December and he is looking to take the line out. He took my central line out and it was a beautiful non event, it simply slipped out without any anguish or problem. Let us hope that this is similar. I also saw Dr Weare which I usually enjoy and he has an idea that a physiotherapist specialising in ultra sound may be beneficial if Dr Marcus approves. He is careful to talk to Dr Marcus before suggesting any treatment as he says Dr Marcus owns the transplant and we are not going to rock the boat.

I forgot to mention it to Dr Weare but my feet are hurting again. Deja vu perhaps.

November 24 – 29

Still the same old slog but I am eating my tiny amounts with a knife and fork at least a semblance of normality. The ultrasound treatment consists of a gel being spread along the shingles tracks and then a nozzle is applied which supplies the ultrasound. The nozzle hurts when it is applied and there is no guarantee of success but it is well worth a try. It will not cure the shingles but could lessen the pain. The real cure will come in due course but I have been waiting for six months now. Please hurry up.

November 30 – December 1

My line is out not without problems. When we went to the hospital it seems that they were not expecting us and it took a little persuasion and a bit of luck to get the operation under way. Both Dr Marcus and Dr Weare said that they could have taken it out, by " just pulling it", what a good job they were not given the chance.

Dr Jameson removed it in the theatre and it had a flap of skin growing into a cusp which was to anchor it. This had to be surgically removed, and I shudder to think what "just pulling it out" would have done to me. I was awake the whole time, and felt nothing, the whole thing went off very well. I found it very hard not to laugh at the clothes worn in the theatre, mine included, they must be used to it.

I also saw the E.N.T. specialist, Mr Ellis, while I was there and he confirms what he said at our last meeting. There is an operation which will bring an immediate improvement. This involves a two man team, one going in through an incision in the neck whilst the other operates in the throat via mirrors. It sounds dreadful but obviously the doctors have been talking to each other and would not recommend that I go ahead with this now. The conclusion is that I have had such a rough time recently that it would be better if I regained my strength first. No arguments from me on that score, it was pleasing that it was the opinion of the doctors that I have had a bad time. It could have been that I was having minor problems but that I was a wimp. At some stage I will have to have the voice sorted out, it is still a whisper. I phoned my employers last week and they thought I was a heavy breather. I cannot work like this, nor can I return to the Bench as chairman like this, so something will have to give.

I am still carrying on with the ultra sound but the shingles is still very sore. I have had many false dawns over this but my revulsion towards food is going and I am eating slightly more. I feel sure that I am on the mend but the key to it all is the eating. I am convinced that once I start to eat I will be fine. Then I will only have to sort the shingles out, repair the Biafra style body, the strength, and the impotence. There is a lovely song by the Commodores which I could adapt, "Three Times a Lady", I could re-title it "Three Times Infertile". The first is the vasectomy, second is the chemo, and third is the impotence brought about by the weakness. We shall overcome.

December 2 – 7

I saw Dr Marcus again and he is very pleased with my progress. The girls who had nursed me were all coming up to say how well I was looking and this made me feel even better. It was very much like the Stanley Holloway monologue, "My word you do look well". There is no need to see Dr Marcus until February so that must be another good sign.

I feel that I have turned the corner at long last on the eating front. I have hardly dared hope as I have had so many set-backs, but I am increasing the variety and the amount, eating with proper plates and with a proper knife and fork. It sounds like toddler training. The total food intake is now possibly 25% of my previous appetite, and by eating more of the "wrong" kind of food, the high calorie stuff, I have pushed my calorie intake over 2000 per day. This means that the dreaded Complan having done the job admirably, has been consigned to the wheelie bin. Never in the history of refuse collection has an item been so willingly donated.

Christmas is rapidly approaching, and whilst I know that I will not be 100%, it is not an ordeal, I am looking forward to it rather than fearing it. It is all coming good.

December 8 – 13

I saw Dr Weare and it is good to keep in touch and to chat over any problems. Every time I see Dr Marcus he writes to Dr Weare and I call in shortly afterwards. He is pleasantly surprised that I am looking so well so quickly and at the fact that my eating has improved so much. We also thought that it would be a good idea to have a flu jab and I felt strangely weak after it. I got a prescription for pain killers but as the side effects are fatigue and liver inflammation, I will not use it. Nothing is going to get in the way of my progress.

I went to see the magistrates before their sitting and the Court clerks, ushers, etc., and they were delighted to see me. I have not had so many cuddles for a long time. It must have been a relief for a prodigal son to return as we have had a horrible year. Out of a bench of 19, there has been my illness, another member with cancer, two ladies had operations, another lost her son and found that her husband was ill, another had a daughter ill, and yet another lost her father. For me to be coming back to fitness was a rare event to dispel the gloom.

I was amazed how tired I was when I returned until I felt the weight of the coat I was wearing. Fit people never give this a thought, but it nearly shattered me.

December 14 – 21

I am still going to my ultrasound sessions but I don't think they are the answer. The shingles still hurt and I still have the pain killing prescription in the drawer and that is where it will stay. My appetite is still increasing slowly but steadily, and I am looking forward to Christmas. One odd thing, at the moment I can drink Guinness but not beer. I have not tried lager, but I never liked boys' beer anyway so I will not bother. Scotch needs to be watered down so I can only take blended. I do not propose to water malt so that will stay where it is for the time being. I heard of a test supposedly given to cocktail barmen. Ask him to serve a malt Scotch and green ginger and if he does sack him.

I have pencilled in returning to the Bench early in the new year but only as a winger, and hope to go back to work in a silent role in Feb/March. I have not worked for Dow Stoker for long but what a terrific bunch of people they are.

The football front is unbelievable. We are having the best season for ages, playing some lovely stuff. I have a sister living in Sunderland who had the sense to marry a Sunderland fanatic and there is a steady flow of newspapers, videos, and books. I hope Jean and Pete realise how much this means to me, and to my boys who receive the material after me. They have not been through a season like this. After drawing with Reading we are top of the league, and are due to play Manchester United in the cup in the New Year.

Years ago when Ian was seven I took him to his first game at Luton. I was determined never to push the boys into football but it made it even sweeter when they chose it themselves. On this particular day Sunderland were having a bad day and when Luton scored their second goal, Ian said to me, "Never mind Dad, it's only a game." The blokes around us were helpless.

December 22 – 26

Christmas Day passed well, I ate more than I had thought possible and had the odd drink or two. Telephone calls from Australia, the North East and Germany, where June's brother lives, really made the day. For the first time in ages I could look forward to the New Year with absolute confidence.

We are trying to arrange a holiday and looking through the travel brochures it looks as if the Canaries, with an average temperature of 72°F, will fit the bill. All that is left is to confirm with Dr Marcus and my G.P. Dr Weare that I am fit enough to go, contact the insurance company to see if they are happy, and we can book. I need some sun on my shingles and after the year June has had it will be marvellous to see her resting.

December 27 – 31

Christmas has passed and there is New Year to come. Being a semi-Geordie, New Year has always meant more than Christmas and now is the time to sit quietly and contemplate the old year and the new. This year it is easy as the old year was the worst of my life so far and the new opens out into getting back into shape and hopefully full fitness.

My resolution for the New Year will be to become normal once again and to contribute something to my family and friends instead of being a burden. I have hated not only my illness but the knowledge that I was not functioning properly either as a father or as a male. It may seem ludicrous but it hurts constantly having to see a wife who you adore having to do things like setting out the bin, opening jars, things that were normally passed to me but no longer.

As far as I am concerned 1995 can sink into its own cesspit, I want nothing more to do with it. The Queen talks about her "Annus Horribilus." Ma'am, yours was a doddle.

Chapter Eight – The Final Come Back

January 1 – 7, 1996

The New Year has started well. We went to Barry and Chris for New Year's Eve, and I was surprised at my stamina as I was still awake and sensible at 2am. Without going into too many details my impotence is a thing of the past. What a good way to start the year.

My weight is still creeping up, it seems to go to a natural barrier, like 8st 13, and sticks there for a while. I have managed to push it over to 9st 1, so another barrier has been breached. Have started doing more on the rowing machine although I suffer the next day. I am eating more both in quantity and variety and I now look forward to meals instead of trying to hide. It is odd that anything tomato-based like baked beans, still revolt me, and I can't manage eggs yet. This apart, everything is great.

Sunderland outplayed Manchester United in the cup, but had to settle for a draw. I may be ever so slightly biased but that was the view shared by all football commentators and including Alex Ferguson who said that they were lucky to draw. I could not make the journey and would have loved to be there but this is what you have sons for, to keep the flag flying. The journey to Manchester is bad from this part of the country and I made an early decision not to go. My sister, however, still managed to get two tickets and my lads were able to go instead. They said it was one of the best days of their lives, very emotional and satisfying. I saw the game of course on T.V. and it was great to see us play so well and hear the complimentary things said about us. There is a brave new year ahead.

January 8 – 10

June rang Dr Marcus and he can see no reason why I can not go abroad providing it is not to anywhere exotic, meaning poor hygiene standards. The insurance company simply want a letter from my G.P. saying that I am clinically well and we can book a holiday. I was concerned about this even though I knew that terminal patients go on holiday, so there had to be a procedure covering illness.

I am aching from the rowing machine but it is far too early to say whether it is doing any good. What I am trying to do now is to push myself a bit more to see how far I can go. I went to Saffron Walden yesterday and drove there which was the first time for over a year. Also I had lunch in a cafe which was also the first time for a year. It should have been a hat – trick as I was supposed to attend a meeting, also the first for a year, but had to cancel it.

My brother Alf was calling to see us, and family comes before meetings. Alf and Eileen have been stalwarts during my illness, spending fortunes on the telephone and calling whenever they were in the area. I will see a fair bit of them as their daughter, my niece Jennifer, is to be married near Redhill, and they are making frequent trips. Jennifer called to see us a while ago and I had just gone to bed exhausted after a visit to Dr Marcus and they would not disturb me. I wish they had.

January 11 – 20

Apart from the shingles, which I think I am making worse with the rowing, things are going well. June noticed that I have been walking trying to keep my arm still because of the shingles pain and it is pulling my right shoulder forward. This is crazy if after all I have been through I make myself deformed.

I was determined to put the missing weight back as muscle and not fat and it appears to be working. The problem is that the right side of my body is noticeably bigger than the left. This is because of the action of the rowing machine which operates with two handles and as I am right handed I tend to favour that side. I will have to do my normal work and then do extra solely on the left side to put this right.

I mentioned my "left sidedness" to Dr Weare when I went to pick up the letter for the insurance company and we ended up having a laugh about it. He asked me how much I was doing on the rowing machine, and I told him, 25. He blanched at this and said that he went to a gym, and he could get nowhere near 25 minutes. I managed to put his mind at rest by telling him that I was doing 25 strokes, not minutes.

After a fair bit of deliberation because I knew June could not come, I went to the Magistrates Dinner on the 12th. I was really pleased that I had made the effort as it was so good to see everyone and to meet the new magistrates who have been appointed since my illness. True, my appetite is not completely back, and my voice is nowhere near normal, but the evening was so satisfying. At one point during the evening the Chairman thanked me for making the effort to attend and everyone stood and applauded. Altogether a very pleasurable, nostalgic and emotional evening.

After a struggle we are booked for Lanzarote, and it should be great, get the sun on my shingles, and the toes in the sand. Alf is coming next week to see Jennifer and is calling to see us. I will accomplish another three "firsts". We are going out for a meal with Alf and Eileen, plus a Governors' meeting at the school, and a drink with Phil Tripp, one of my magisterial colleagues. He has had to retire on reaching the age of 70, and his experience and knowledge is going to waste. We are all aware of the dangers of letting people go on too long but surely a magistrate, on reaching 70, could renew each year and carry on as long as the fitness lasts. Judges are allowed to go on, I feel that we should also.

January 21 – 31

I attended the Governors meeting at Leventhorpe which was the first for over a year. They gave me a round of applause when they realised who it was under all the scarves and cap. Quite moving, as they have kept in touch through the Chairman who has called to see me often including the times when I was at my lowest ebb. It must have been a bit funny as well. There are various meetings and when the other Governors asked how I was doing, Roger, the Chairman, would say that I have gastritis. Next time it would be shingles, then pneumonia and so on.

The only problem was that it was sleeting by the time I got out and I got to the car absolutely freezing and it took me over an hour to thaw out. I just can't take this weather it is the worst I can remember. It was the same when we went out for a meal with Alf and Eileen. The pub was cold and the walk back was beyond description.

I went back to the magistrates session and was foiled. I only saw one person who I had already seen plus two new ones who I had never seen before.

I have been back to see Dr Weare and I always feel better when I come out. He reached the final of a competition to find the most caring G.P. in the country, it is easy to see why. My voice is just as weak and I still have to shout to get any volume but the odd bass/baritone is breaking through. Dr Weare says it is a sign that the vocal cords are being used more and it is the start of the voice coming back.

Weight now 9st 4.

February 1 – 5

Looking forward to Lanzarote but there are signs of unease, hopefully imagination. I still have a constant shingles pain and muscle ache from the exercise but now I have headaches and my eyes hurt. I can only hope that this is a temporary blip, as my appetite is getting worse.

Something else I hope is a temporary blip is the football. Since the magnificent displays in the cup ties we have done nothing. We have just lost 3-0 to Wolves and are down to 5th in the table, the promotion race is slipping away. One thing should be stopped if the F.A had any guts at all.

We were due to play Norwich on the Saturday then Manchester United in the cup replay on the following Wednesday. Along came the great God Television and we ended up playing on Sunday and Tuesday. Thank you, money bags, we are really grateful, especially as we lost both games. Football belongs to the people not television moguls, "Can we have our game back please?"

I hate the present set up. The Premier League was set up by the greedy big boys who could not care less if smaller clubs go to the wall. The thrill of looking at the results has largely gone as the games are now played to suit the T.V. schedules and not the fans. Whenever big money comes into a sport the sport always change, and always for the worse.

February 6 – 8

It may be nerves, but I have had diarrhoea for 2 days before going to Lanzarote. It seems to be all right now, and it will not stop us going. Let us get away from this abominable weather, let me take my shingles to the sun and load up on food as my weight is starting to go down. It could be the diarrhoea or the replacement of a bit of fat with muscle, but I will need to watch it.

February 9 – 16

We always have good holiday weather, it had to change sometime. There was a freak weather system over the Canaries and it was perishing cold almost all the time. I had to ask for an extra blanket and lay in bed fully clothed and shivering during the worst days. The maids cleaned the cooker with water, which meant that the lights were fused every day. The hotel was poor, the food only moderate and my diarrhoea got worse for three days.

I wondered if this was the food or my old problems coming back, but thankfully it was neither. It was an awful bug I picked up in England before I left. It was good to know that I could pick up normal problems and shake them off, my bodily defences must be working well. The wind on my chest was hard to bear and it was freezing cold, but at least it meant that when we returned home, the weather was slightly warmer, and not the usual shock to the system. This is the first holiday I have never been in the water, which was a pity as I had been looking forward to it. We enjoyed each other's company free from distractions, but the holiday was a write off.

The voice is improving slowly and I now have three voices, sultry whisper, Dalek and Donald Duck. I have no control over which one is currently in use, which caused me a spot of bother in Court. I had to tell a defendant that he would be placed on probation but that if he did not respond, the only thing left was prison. I switched into pure Dalek, and it must have sounded hilarious, particularly the "do you understand?" bit at the end. It is just like when my voice broke all those years ago. I hope that the other things happen as well this time, I seem to remember walking around like Max Wall for ages.

February 17 – 25

At last I am convinced that my voice is getting better. It is still weak but is coming back to my normal timbre and it looks like being yet another long job before it is completely right. It is going in the right direction, so any good news is welcome. The shingles is still bad and now I have another seemingly minor problem which is causing me unexpected grief.

During the chemo sessions, the nail beds were killed on my big toes. They are now growing out but I have a ridge of dead nail being pushed out by the new nail underneath. This ridge is a bit loose, and catches against socks, rubs when I walk and generally tries to make life difficult.

The outside world is going mad. By all accounts the I.R.A. is starting up again, and it is strange why they ever agreed to a cease fire in the first place. No doubt the Americans will now bow to the Irish vote and support them like last time. I had the misfortune to watch part of the British Pop Awards and it left me amazed. People were making obscene gestures and using appalling language.

Why do we have to put up with this behaviour? Why can they not be arrested or at least ejected? These louts smash up aircraft and hotel rooms and nothing is done. It is about time the law was used to curb these people. At the very least we could prevent loons like Michael Jackson coming over here to peddle his banal wailings. The world has been taken over by these people and it is time we got it back.

I am getting to hate the bowing down of everyone to others whose sole asset seems to be the possession of money; quality or manners are not prized any more.

February 26 – 28

Went to see Dr Marcus and drove through to Cambridge. He was delighted with my progress and said that he expected to see me three times a year from now on. This is the best news as this is the maximum he allows between appointments, so things must be almost as good as they can be. All this is on the understanding that the tests he did do not show anything odd. There is no reason at all why they should, but I know that I will be very impatient until I hear.

After my examination, when I am getting dressed Dr Marcus talks to June until I am ready and I think that this talk is very valuable. I may decide to send her through in future and save me the trouble of going. The muscles at the top of my arms are going mad, obviously in driving they are being used for the first time in over a year.

February 29 – March 10

What a week this has been, I have deliberately extended myself, and have been to court twice, school three times, a Committee meeting and a cocktail party. I ended up very tired, but I handled it, and was very pleased.

Sunderland are doing well, still 2nd in the League and looking a very solid, reliable and consistent side.

March 11 – 14

Still no news of my tests and I am getting jumpy, not because I am expecting bad news, but I am simply impatient. My niggles continue, and I expect they will for some time yet, but the appetite is about 95% of what it was.

I have arranged to go up to the North East next month and will take in the Charlton game at Roker Park. The way things are going this may be the Championship decider. We have won the last 6 games, and have not lost since February 3.

I found out that we are to become grandparents which is wonderful news and may mean more Australia trips than we had planned. This terrific news was shattered however with news of the Dunblane tragedy. A deranged man broke into a school and killed 16 tots and their teacher. There is nothing in life, no training or experience, which can prepare ordinary people for things like this.

The photographs of the children were published and in many cases the photographer had captured shots that all parents try for but few attain. There is the little girl who has just realised her power over her father and the little lad who has just thought of some mischief. Lovely photographs, lovely children destroyed in a sick evil moment. I felt sick, I dread to think what their relatives went through. I would hope that everyone not involved will stay away, including, or perhaps especially, counsellors and leave these shattered people to repair themselves.

March 15 – 22

I have heard from Dr Marcus, and I am now officially in remission. At first I have to admit to being a little disappointed, as a layman I prefer the word cured. Completely professional as always, he would not put anything in a letter which was not absolutely correct. He did say in layman's language that things are now going extremely well and that I have absolutely nothing to worry about, so I won't. I suppose after five years I will be rated as cured but by then I will have forgotten all about this last year.

There seems little point in carrying on with these notes so often either, as not much is happening now. What started off as a few jottings to send to Andie have expanded and I hope they are of some use to someone. When I was diagnosed I wanted to speak to someone who had previously had myeloma but was unable to. Even later, when the transplant was over, I was still trying to find people with personal experience of how long the anorexia and the shingles would last but again I was unable to. If I think it is good enough I may offer this record to CancerBacup, as myeloma is so uncommon it may be that they still are short of information on a personal level, not purely clinical.

It might make grisly bedtime stories for my grandchild, although Wizard Reid and his wondermen is probably a better one. We are firmly at the top of the league and look like going up with points to spare.

Chapter Nine – Reflections

I am still not fully fit, but I feel my strength returning. This does not mean necessarily that I will get back to the same physical well being as I was before. The amount of chemo I have had and the various reactions to the drugs must inevitably leave a mark. Add to this the fact that Anno Domini is a constant threat. It may well be that a reduced level of fitness is the best I can hope for but I will certainly not give up easily.

There are physical changes and it is too early to tell if they will be permanent. The blessed shingles has not abated at all, although every one of the doctors has said that it will take its own time, but that it will go away. My voice is improving and for a part of each day it is normal but also each day it gets tired and I end up croaking and, strangely, coughing. As I still labour on the rowing machine, what pass for muscles ache, but I am putting weight back on my shoulders and arms and I can see myself eventually returning to my previous build.

My appetite, for so long a source of anguish and despair to everyone, but especially to June and myself, is almost completely back to normal. I am eating everything having taken a while to conquer eggs and tomato. The only difference is that previously I liked everything, but now there are things that I am not too fond of, although I still eat them. I am also eating slowly, but this could be a consequence of having a restricted jaw movement. The hinge on my jaw does not seem to want to open fully and this slows me down. Possibly this could have happened during my liquid diet and it may come back.

My eyes are easily irritated after my bout of conjunctivitis, and feel tight from time to time. Almost unbelievably, my head is smaller and this might be causing pressure on the eyes. I put on a hat I had not worn since before my illness and it slipped down over my ears, and my hat size is now two sizes smaller. I hate hats and have no intention of using one when my period of sensitivity is over but it is important now. When I forget my hat and go out in the sun, my face comes out in blotches, and my eyes start to itch. I was warned that prolonged chemo damages the teeth. A filling has dropped out and I had to go to my dentist full of trepidation. He simply replaced it and said that my teeth were in really good condition so I seem to have escaped one of the side effects, it is about time.

All of the above I expect will fade over time, and only then will I be able to tell if the treatment and side effects have left a permanent reminder. It may be that I have gone back to my previous metabolism, as even with my prodigious eating habits, I have just got up to 10 stone (21 May). For years I infuriated colleagues who shared lunches and Bank Dinners by eating twice as much as them and not putting on an ounce.

June thinks that my hearing is not as sharp as it was but our G.P. thinks this could be due to nerve damage and will get better in time. My voice is now almost back to normal after nerve damage, so I am hopeful. The downside is that recovery from nerve problems seems to take forever. What I believe has happened, although I hope I am wrong, is my brain is not as good. Certainly my memory has lapses and I do not seem to be able to grasp things as quickly as I once did but again this may recover in time. It may even be the advancing years, but I will not accept that until I am forced to. I see this recovery not so much as becoming well again, but of reaching my prime.

One thing I am sure about is that I will never have cancer again. It is the same logic as the man who was terrified of flying as he had a fixation about a bomb being on the aircraft. His solution was to take one on himself. The odds on an aircraft carrying a bomb are a million to one, the odds on two separate bombs are 50 million to one. I think that about my cancer. Apparently one third of people contract cancer, and I have had mine and got over it. This must reduce the chance of me getting it again, similar to the second bomb. It means that I can carry on my life now certain that cancer will never again rear its ugly head.

In some ways I seem to have changed. It would be difficult to stay exactly the same in view of my experiences over the last 18 months or so, I have been confronted with situations which for me were alarming. My attitude to money has softened, it was previously typically ex-bank manager. I have resisted selling shares or realising investments, but now if we need something, we get it. It may well be that all this trouble has done me good.

I seem to be less robust than before. Physically I am much lighter and weaker, but I am not as strong mentally and tend to worry a lot. My sleeping habits are curtailed by the pain of the shingles and when I am awake at four in the morning the old nightmares are still lurking if I am not careful. My thoughts at this time of the morning would provide Edgar Allen Poe with material for half a dozen novels.

I will never forget the days I was racked in agony before the shingles showed itself and I was allowed treatment for the gastritis. I was in deep despair and looking at life now after that experience gives a different slant. That gave me a new perspective on what is important in life. What people class as important has largely been put there by the advertising moguls, new cars, fashions, etc. and it takes something like an illness to show just how minor these things are. When I see youngsters with caps turned round and wearing shirts below their jackets, it makes me smile. I smile partly because they look so unbelievably silly, but mostly because the drive to be "with it" is so shallow and banal and has no true importance whatever.

During the time I was at my lowest ebb I heard a discussion on the subject of the living will. The dreadful condition I was in gave me an early insight to old age and infirmity, and it is not a pleasant prospect. The living will, if ever it is made legal, will allow people to specify in advance how much treatment they want in certain circumstances. I could not face the prospect of Alzheimer's, or a severe stroke leaving me with no idea who I was. I would be more than happy to sign a document now preventing the doctors from keeping me alive in those circumstances. I have been enough of a burden recently, enough is enough.

I think I am more relaxed and more patient than previously, but only with peoples foibles and behaviour. Before, when I disagreed with someone, it coloured my judgement of the whole person. Now I am able to see that as part of a whole raft of opinions and a realisation that it may be me who is wrong. How does the quotation go? – "Think, I beseech thee in the bowels of Christ to consider that ye may be wrong." Oliver Cromwell and me both, but I think that I am now more placid and more forgiving. Opinions, even faults I can now accept far more easily than before. Another quotation, "If two people agree on everything, one of them is not necessary."

My illness has made me more tolerant with people, but I still get annoyed at things which are simply not important and which are made out to be so. A serious illness is a perfect way of giving a perspective of what is truly important and what is simply dross. I have seen fashion experts on T.V. waxing lyrical on how two and three year old girls should be given the opportunity to wear designer dresses at £200 each. The world is full of millions of people dying of starvation, easily preventable diseases and in wars. This is truly important, and yet we have fashion experts discussing at length what colour will be popular this year. What a shallow outlook these people must have.

I have already expressed my opinion on fortune tellers but just as facile is the glorification of nonsense in the media. The goings on in the soaps take over from reality. Politicians jump in on the act be saying how wonderful the soaps are in a thinly disguised attempt to be seen as a "common man". It only needs a character in a soap to be pregnant and the T. V. studios are full of people earnestly discussing the implications. What is our society becoming?

Tell me if you will that such things are a harmless diversion from everyday life and I will accept that but please do not pretend that they have quality or that they are in the slightest way important. If nothing else, my illness has taught me that it is people who are important, and I think our society is moving away from that, to its detriment. The news has just been announced that Jaymee Bowen, of "Child B" fame has died. It makes me feel really sad, although even living in the same village, I had never met her. The odds were always stacked against her and she certainly gave it all she had but regrettably it was not be. What makes me cross is the way the "informed opinion " pundits are using her life and death as a stick to hit the N.H.S. and the Government with.

When I became ill, it took me some while to reconcile the different ways people dealt with the news. A few avoided both the news and me, but it was rare most of my friends and family surprised me with the depth of their feelings. This may seem odd and it is certainly difficult to explain, one of the hardest things to rationalise in the whole experience. To my family I was a husband, father, brother, son in law or whatever and for them to have deep feelings is more understandable. One strange thing is that my mother-in-law, ostensibly a practical Yorkshire-woman, has said recently that in the early days she felt odd talking to me and would not ask how I was in case I had bad news, or in case she upset me. She did not visit as she did not want to add to the work load and, in any case, coming from the North East is a fair trek.

My friends have been amazing, and have been a great help to both of us all the way through. It has been very difficult to understand the depth of their feelings for me which they demonstrated on many occasions. They clearly did feel deeply and I find it very hard to come to terms with that. Put bluntly, I found it hard to see what it was in me that caused such a reaction. I can only say that looking at myself over the years, I have never had a very good opinion of myself and therefore found it hard to understand how others could feel so much. The fact that they do sustained me in the dark times, and it is something I will always be grateful for, and feel humble about.

Perhaps during the advice sessions before the treatment starts more should be said about finance. I know that Gilda Bass talks about money but concentrates on income and help available from the various Departments. We were all right on that score, but I was not prepared for the costs during my illness and recovery. The loss of income for 18 months is obvious, but the miles to and from Cambridge, and the savage depreciation on our car is something I had not taken into account. New clothes, different foods which in many cases had to be thrown out as I could not eat them, there are many and varied costs which I would not have thought possible. While I was ill, there has been no decoration at home and now it has to be done all together. As I am still unable to tackle things like ceilings, we have to get professionals in and they are not cheap.

The clothing side amazed me as I had thought only of waist sizes, never dreaming that everything is now smaller, hands, feet, even my head. New things have to be bought in the full knowledge that when I get back to my normal size they will be useless. It may be fine for people who like shopping for clothes but I detest it. I hold various records for choosing new clothes, like sports jacket two minutes, shoes four minutes, simply to get out of shops as soon as possible.

There must be an opening for a self employed garment fondler. Almost without exception people go into shops on Saturday mornings and grab hold of a garment sleeve at the shoulder, and slowly slide their hands down to the cuff. Heaven knows why they do that but the garment fondler could offer to do it on behalf of all their neighbours and friends and let them stay in bed, in exchange for a small fee. There must be some primeval urge that forces people to go into shops but it is one that thankfully has evaded me.

When I read my notes, I still can not quite accept that it all happened to me. It proves that although a serious illness can drag you down to despair and beyond you still come out of the other side. I have almost taken up where I left off on gardening, which I enjoy, and generally pottering about the garden and kitchen, which I also enjoy. Time will tell whether my faculties return undiminished but they are well on the way and I am confident that they will.

As long as I live, I will be profoundly grateful for the staff at Addenbrooke's Ward 10, my consultant and the staff at The Evelyn and my GPs. They have all in their own way been magnificent. My family and friends have been without equal and it is hard to overestimate their input in my recovery. In the black times hardly a day passed without at least one of my friends calling. Barry and Chris, Bert and Janet, Judy and Jim, Pat and Ken, they all played a significant and irreplaceable part in my recovery. Jane and David, though living miles away, played their part, and the notes of encouragement they sent me were so helpful.

The world wide net I referred to earlier tightened around me and sustained me in the bad times. Andie and Steve, Carole and Graeme from Australia, Harold and his family from Germany, Reg and Shelagh all played a part. My sister called from Milton Keynes, but she is the only one in the area. Alf and Eileen made many trips from the North East, and spent many hours on the telephone as did my other sister Jean and her husband Peter. They have a business in Sunderland which demands their presence and yet they made time to visit and contact me. The list goes on.

June has been a tower of strength, a five foot colossus who dragged me through the bleak times, and there were many. I am now on four monthly visits to my consultant and as my recovery continues, the acute memory is fading and in time will fade still more. I will keep this record to remind me of how it was and renew my gratitude to all involved. The personal relationships are the only good thing to come out of all of this. My illness and recovery has brought me into contact with many wonderful people but I am sure they will not be annoyed if I would have preferred that none of it had ever happened.

As a final note on non medical matters, Sunderland did win the League and will be up with the other big boys next season. Already the media are saying that we will come straight down again, which I dispute, and that we will need to strengthen the team, which of course is true. At least we were promoted without spending obscene amounts of money. It is inevitable the way things are going that football will suffer. The colossal amounts of money being paid out can only mean higher admission charges and when fathers can no longer afford to take their sons to a game we are on the slippery slope. Very soon, because of the huge costs, many clubs will go part-time, or non league and then where will the players come from? In the meantime, let the supporters enjoy the success that is long overdue. Lots of our fans go to the away games to places like Oldham and Southend who get small gates and are grateful for the extra 4000 people who make the pilgrimage. Sunderland supporters must be among the most ardent in the country and, coming from a traditionally depressed area, they are entitled to enjoy it to the full, as I intend to do.

Chapter Ten – Slowly But Surely

I had decided not to take notes as often, as nothing startling is happening, things are developing certainly slowly, hopefully, surely. It seems almost ungrateful to mention the problems I am having now as I must compare my present state to what I was like only months ago. It seems incredible that at one time, I had an extension wire in the living room so that I could answer the telephone if June was out, but I was not strong enough to lift the receiver off the cradle. I had to bend down to it and knock it off so I could speak. Comparing those times to the present seems like another world and another person. Even so, I still have things that annoy me and stop me from improving further.

The shingles pain is with me all of the time but varying in severity. It still is enough to prevent me getting much exercise and on bad nights much sleep, creating a vicious circle which is difficult to break. Shortly after my transplant, my tear ducts virtually packed in, causing me to have eye drops very often, which I hated. Now, I get conjunctivitis easily and it is a nuisance. Not only that, if I am in the car and the air vents are on my eyes become sore and bloodshot. I promise I am not whining, but I now try to think of myself as normal and things like that would aggravate any normal person so it seems that I can't win. When my doctors discuss my shingles they call it by the proper name, and at first I thought it was another new problem.

I drive, but derive almost no pleasure from it. The roads seem to be far busier and it is going to be a long time before I get my confidence and timing back. We had to attend the wedding of my niece, who luckily for me was getting married at Redhill. I drove the car to Gatwick where we were staying, and it was by far the longest I had driven for two years. It was a great occasion for me as I was able to see all my family who came down from the North-East and the wedding went off superbly. Jennifer betrayed her Sunderland traditions by marrying a rabid Leeds supporter but, nevertheless, Kevin is a really nice bloke. This animosity dates from the days when Leeds were playing their 'strong aggressive' football and in one particular game at Roker Park, they were truly disgraceful. If Leeds played Newcastle in the F.A. Cup Final, a lot of Sunderland fans would be shouting for Newcastle.

I managed the drive and we got there safely but my shoulders and arms were very sore and stiff the next day. I had a swim in the small but very warm pool and was very pleased with myself, but clearly I have a long way to go. It was great to see the families together particularly the youngsters who see each other rarely. I thought about the average of 2.2 children per family and out of our family it has just about worked out. We have two sons and a daughter, my brother Alf has one son and two daughters and my sisters Jean and Margarita have one son each.

My family have only been on the same continent once in recent years and now we are to see another one go to Australia. Ian has delayed until he was convinced that I was recovered and obtained his working visa with only weeks to go. He is off down under for a year and although we will miss him, what a great opportunity it is. At the same age, it would have been unthinkable for us to have gone on a trip like that. The thought of giving up a good job was bad enough but the cost in the 60's of a flight to Australia was horrendous. When I worked as an economist, we worked prices out in multiples of how long a skilled worker would have to pay for various commodities. At that time our mythical skilled worker would have needed to work for a few months to pay for the air fare, now it will be just over a week. Good luck to Ian, but it now means that we have three of the family in England, and two in Australia; the ratio will worsen later on in the year when our grandchild appears. Andie is fit as a fiddle, so we are all looking forward to it.

I am struggling on, still weak as I can not get much exercise because of the pain from the shingles, or to dignify it with the proper name, post herpetic neuralgia. It was very bad when the weather was cold and I blamed that, but now that it is warm, there is little or no improvement. I am still being obstinate and refusing the pills I have been offered. My G.P. has given me a prescription and I can have the pills any time I want but I am still resisting, I think I have had all the pills I ever want. I am not being brave, or entering into martyrdom, but as long as I can stand the pain I will carry on.

It is a nuisance, though, with Paul's graduation coming up and obviously we want to go to Hull for the ceremony. He finished up with a 2.2, known to all as a Desmond which is very good in the circumstances. After an abortive work placement he went to Australia for the third year and it must have been very hard to come back and pick up the pieces. I just had to grit my teeth and go, as the worst thing for me is being in a car, and I could not take the wheel much. I am not giving up but I still feel ashamed that I am not pulling my weight.

On the football front, we have bought Tony Coton, Alex Rae, and Niall Quinn, so that should help us although Peter Reid is supposed to have £10 million to spend. Talking of figures like this is immoral when half the world is starving. I hate this Premier League and everything that goes with it. It was started by the greedy clubs who think of nothing but themselves, encouraged by SKY, who are backed by Murdoch; it was doomed from the start. Already, players are being paid £40,000 plus per week, the local players are being squeezed out, supporters are being fleeced by unscrupulous clubs changing strips three times in a season, it is already out of control. I have said it before, when big money comes into a sport, the sport changes, and always for the worse.

Even the Olympic games are so besmirched with the Great God Dollar that it is hardly worth watching. Synchronised swimming was bad enough, now apparently we are to have ballroom dancing. The soft porn, or beach volley ball as it is sometimes known, is ludicrous. If anyone doubts that it is soft porn, just think how successful it would be if the players were 20 st. each and wore overalls, instead of lovely girls in skimpy bikinis. It should go back to the Olympic ideal of an athletic meeting, and nothing else.

As we move into September, Sunderland are sitting comfortably in the middle of the league, I am more than happy with that. I will need to go up to Roker Park this season as it is the last season before we move into our evidently magnificent new stadium. At present I could not face the drive but we are arranging a holiday and there is always the hope that it will put me right. We have a holiday insurance policy which is in force all the year round but I will have to make sure that they are happy. I was pleased that they were willing to leave it to my consultant and G.P. and armed with a letter stating that I am clinically well. At last I can go to the travel agent with confidence.

We are going with our friends Barry and Chris, who were stalwarts during the worst parts of my illness and we were able to compromise. They like to go to the same place most of the time but our choice is to go to a different place each time, We decided to go to Minorca and it mostly went very well. The first week went very well, provided we were sheltered from the wind but I could not believe the change then. We were caught outside when the wind got up and I worried Barry and Chris visibly. I am very good at disguising when I am in pain, but this time the wind was almost hurricane level, and freezing cold and I was not far from collapsing.

After this everyone stayed in the hotel and it was simply a matter of surviving. We were due to go home in three days and people were offering to buy our tickets. One thing I was tempted to do was something which would have caused ructions. There were Bingo sessions run by a Belgian and I was tempted to tell him how the English play the game. Things like Kelley's Eye, No 4, All the fours, 21, Clickety click No 5, the place would have been in turmoil. The wind took the felt roof off the extension, the rain was pouring through the windows, altogether a thoroughly miserable experience. One new thing for me, I tried out a new drink, a Lamumba. It is liberal portions of rum and chocolate, and it is a very pleasant taste, and the effect sneaks up, so it has to be watched. Thank you Patrice, you have named a drink, not much for a life's work. At least it tended to show that my neuralgia was made worse by my clothes pressing against my back at 60 mph in freezing cold. What happens is that it knocks my confidence when I am forced to face the fact that I am not as well as I pretend and that I still have some way to go.

Shortly after we got back from Minorca, it was time for my visit to Dr. Marcus, and he was pleased to see how well I was looking, which always helps. The results of the tests take about two weeks and invariably I get jumpy towards the end. I am sure that everything will be fine, as is Dr. Marcus, but I can not help worrying. It is just another example of my lack of confidence and at times a fragile state of mind. Not a bit robust, it is just as well that I am pretty good at disguising it.

We spent our time counting the days of Andie's pregnancy, she is still perfectly fit, and getting impatient. Steve managed to fax us with the news but with the time difference we were not sure if the baby was born on November 8th or 9th. We have our first grandchild and everything is fine, in fact they were out for a walk when the baby was three days old. She is called Emily, which is a relief, there are many Australian names which we would have cringed at. I can't imagine a little girl with a name like Bluey, or Kylie, it makes me shudder. The great news is that Andie and Steve are going to bring Emily to see us early in the New Year, it would have been nice for Christmas, but that would have been too early for the babe.

This puts a bit of pressure on me, as I must be as fit as I can for their visit and the outcome is that I have succumbed, and have started taking a course of tablets. It bothers me, as I have no wish to be on tablets for the rest of my life but I feel that I must give it a try. It is a good end to the year, Christmas went all right, Paul starts work in the New Year, Sunderland are holding a place in the middle of the table despite an unprecedented run of serious injuries. Roll on 1997.

I can not be sure if the pills I am taking are having any effect as I always have good days and bad days, so there is no pattern to look at. It is my visit to Dr Marcus at the end of the month and maybe he will be able to suggest something. My feet, which started the whole thing off are much improved, so I saw a podiatrist although I dread going to see any kind of an 'ist'. In the event, he thought that they were not too bad and gave me a pair of orthopaedic insoles and after I used them for a while things were much better. In the meantime, we have met little Emily and what an absolute knockout she is. After a 25 hour journey from Sydney, being bundled up in clothing for the first time in her life, and the car journey from Heathrow, she smiled at everyone who held her, what a little peach. Shortly afterwards, we had arranged a party in the North East for the family in the North to meet her and straight back South to another party, for Andie's friends to meet her. She carried on where she had left off, smiling at everyone, she obviously knows the score at three months. After the trip up North and back I was sore and in pain most of the time and was on edge in case Andie realised. Emily beat me hands down.

At the end of the month we had to go to Cambridge to see Dr Marcus and the idea was for all of us to go on to Cambridge, but Emily asserted her authority. It was a foul day, and she had to be wrapped up and she wouldn't have it. She stiffened her arms and made it hard to dress her, we decided it was not worth the effort. Dr Marcus commented on how well I looked, as did Linda Mills, his Sister, and as always this made me feel better. He did say, however, that it was about time we had another try at the neuralgia, and referred me to a specialist, so here we go again.

I went to see Dr Wilkinson, also at Cambridge, and after checking every moving part, and a few that weren't, he suggested doubling the dosage of the pills I was taking, and also to try out a TENS machine. Luckily June had heard of this device and I was willing to try anything, and I arranged to borrow one from our local hospital. The idea of it is to block the messages from the nervous system to the brain and suppress the pain message. Dr Wilkinson told me that the shingles I had has left me with a severely damaged nerve band, and more significantly that he would be unable to cure it but would hope to ease it. I had suspected this for a long time and if I can get it 'putupwithable' to invent a new word, I will have to settle for that.

The only problem is that no-one seems to know much about these strange machines except that they are used in hospitals, and patients do gain relief from pain by using them. Their official name is Transcutaneous Electrical Nerve Stimulation machines, so they should be good with a name like that. I had no idea how long to leave the thing on for so using my famous 'bull at a gate' technique, I left it on for hours at a time. The pads had to be covered with some kind of green gloop which increased the sensation and then were secured by surgical tape on to my skin and very soon I started to dread taking them off. Added to this was the fact that I could never be sure if it was doing any good. There was an improvement, but as I was increasing the pills in stages it might have been that. After a few weeks, I couldn't stand the ravages the tape was wreaking on my skin and stopped for a week.

I was by then taking double the amount of tablets I had taken previously but, as the week wore on, the pain increased, therefore the TENS machine was working. As the pain was getting worse, I was getting more and more depressed, but from another front, the football. Sunderland have been sliding down the League for some weeks and now have a glorious chance to push themselves clear by beating Southampton at home. In the event we played with only one forward and lost. I had the feeling then that we were going down and with the pain I was in, I was to use an old English expression, 'In the slough of despond'. It reminds me of a prosecutor we had in Court, who was very relaxed in his approach, and used to come out with some lovely phrases. On a day during which the local girls school sent some senior girls round to see how a court works, we had a case of indecent exposure. The prosecutor asked the witness, "Was the member turgid, or was it flaccid?" What a lovely word, flaccid.

I digress, back to the TENS machine. I decided to buy one and was able to go to Woodford and actually talk to the people who made them and were as knowledgeable as anyone. As my pain was chest, side and back, they suggested that I have one with two channels, and therefore could tackle two sites at once. Also, I got some self adhesive pads and this made me more confident altogether. I then had to experiment with the machine and to find out for myself how often to use it. Taking the pads off was bliss compared to the tape and by trial and error, I hope to find a great improvement.

The last weekend of April, we went with Barry and Chris to the Lake District, one of my favourite haunts when I was a young lad. On various occasions I spent four or five weeks there and it rained every day. After our experience in Minorca, I was determined that they understood the vagaries of the climate and should be prepared. In the event, of course, the weather was glorious, and I even managed a walk round Grasmere, which although not very arduous, was my first walk for three years.

All this time we were running up to the General Election, and my view was that we had a bad Government, but that it could be better than anything else on offer. Every previous Labour administration had ended in tears, and although the old die hard socialists are being kept under wraps, I am nervous. I remember the last time, with inflation at 26.9 percent, unemployment spiralling, production falling, and everything about us falling to pieces, it is a worry. Against that the present Government presents a very harsh face to all but the successful and that does not sit well with me. Have they forgotten Iain MacLeod so soon? 'There must be a level below which no- one is allowed to fall, and above that everyone should succeed according to his abilities'. I wish all governments would stick to this. If Labour do get in, and it looks likely, I can only hope for the best. Tony Blair does not look like a Prime Minister, or sound like a Prime Minister; I only hope he acts like one.

Chapter 11 – I'm Still Standing

Two days later, still experimenting with my machine, I could only drive part of the way to Sunderland for an afternoon of pure nostalgia. There is a warning not to drive with it connected , strange when they say there are absolutely no side effects. It was the game against Everton and was the very last League game at Roker Park before demolition takes place. I sat there remembering where I used to stand when I was nine years old, and watching over the years players like Shackleton, Ford, Hurley, Clough, the first game of Montgomery, and from other teams, people like Doherty, Mannion, Lawton, Finney, Matthews, Law, Charlton, the list is endless. I fear we will never see their like again, especially if the worst excesses of the Premier League are not curbed, and they won't be.

The nostalgia flooded back, from the time I was allowed to go on my own when I must have been ten years old. There was a pipe running the length of the fence at the Fulwell End, and the little ones used to climb on to that, which was the only way to see. Feet firmly planted on the pipe, hanging on to the top of the fence, we had a great view. In a few years I was too big for that but there was a large step half way down the terracing, and that became my home for the next few years until I reached man's estate. It was almost a rite of passage in our family that the men went to the Roker End, and so it was with me. The crowds were massive and my place was under the pylon at the left hand side going into the ground and was for many years.

I have always preferred to stand and absorb the full atmosphere and I had my education expanded to the point where certainly my mother would have been horrified. The chants used to start at one of the open ends, and football fans were never known for decorum. They were usually coarse and in remarkably bad taste. If there was a visiting player or manager who was flamboyant, like Malcolm Allison with his Fedora and cigar, the crowd may judge that he could do with being taken down a peg a two. He would be given a version of 'Who the Effin?' If anyone wonders how a football crowd all start to sing or chant at the same time, I have the answer. They don't. It builds up gradually, as in 'Who the Effin?' It is sung to the tune of Men of Harlech, and the first line, 'Who the Effin?' may be started by 50 people, by the time the line is repeated, there may be 500 singing. The line 'Who the Effing hell are you?' goes out from many thousands of throats and when the final repeat of 'Who the Effing hell are you?' is reached there may well be half the stadium involved. Men of Harlech has given birth to a few football chants that I know of. A few women police officers have beaten a hasty retreat with scarlet faces when faced with the refrain 'Get your tits out for the lads'. Earthy, crude and in bad taste it may be, but I spent an awful lot of my growing up on those terraces. Even now, although updated the same kind of humour is heard. At my last visit to Sunderland, a loudspeaker announcement asked 'Would the owner of a Lada, Registration E——', the rest was drowned in roars of 'Who the hell's going to own up to that?'

We won the very last game 3-0, and the players did a lap of honour then they stopped and the small figure of Peter Reid came out of the tunnel, and the whole place erupted. I had my hand on the rail in front of me and it was vibrating with the noise. Luckily the club allowed cameras into the ground and I have a picture of the last kick of the last ball of the very last match at Roker Park, ever. I will never forget it. Very sad, but the new ground is said to be one of the best in Europe, but that is another day. I only hope that we stay up, otherwise the biting comment I heard will be more real. The new pitch is currently being spread with manure, the comment is obvious. One puzzle has been cleared up. I have wondered for some time what would happen to the turf on which deceased supporters have had their ashes scattered. The answer is that those areas are to be taken up and relaid in the new ground.

My TENS machine is far more pleasant to use than the old one but I am still not sure I am getting the best out of it yet. I am hurting but then I have spent a lot of time in and out of cars and this is the worst thing I can do. We changed the car some while ago purely to get a car with power steering and although this helps me, I find concentration difficult and sitting uncomfortable. Because of this I get no pleasure from driving but hopefully this will improve.

The new Government have been in for two weeks now, and they are entitled to be cocky after the unbelievable trouncing they gave the Conservatives. It is clearly the honeymoon period as yet but everything they have done so far appears to have a humane side to it, perhaps it is a good thing that they have the chance to succeed. Certainly the way the Conservatives behaved before the election they deserved to lose, but a few good men like Rifkind were swept away along with the dross. The 'sleaze' accusations just will not go away. My own view may seem harsh but if these people are guilty and it is an imprisonable offence then they should go to prison.

I have started to feel ill at ease with the pills I am taking, I seem to be getting too many of the stated side effects. Certainly, I can not concentrate, there is a loss of libido, general tiredness, and depression. I have been back to Dr Weare and he is taking me off the pills gradually over the space of four weeks, and then let the TENS machine do the job. As the pills are reducing and leaving my system I am feeling no extra pain so it seems that my machine is working. I am now cutting down the time I spend on it and suspect that the optimum will be slightly under two hours in the morning and then take it off for the day.

A newspaper article struck me as absurd, if I may digress. Film companies are in financial trouble as the stars are demanding perks which are very expensive. I can offer this solution, and will expect a fat consultancy fee for it – Say No.

At this late stage, I have learned about a myeloma conference in Scotland in July. It is ironic that I could find little information when I needed it and now everything I needed is there. We have decided to go to this conference and make a holiday out of it. The Scots could not get over the weather, for once it was glorious. I think it is important for people like me, who have been through the treatment, to attend, just to show any new patients the final result. It did me a lot of good for people to ask who the patient is, I must look well. The only problem I had was the format. The range of experts attending was very impressive but they all had prepared their 'spiel' individually. This meant that every one started off with the statement that no cure had been found and that mortality rates had hardly altered. By lunch time I was starting to feel like the character in Stanley Holloway's monologue, 'My word you do look queer!' Myeloma is still described as an illness with no cure but I would rather not be reminded. There were a few reminders of how nasty myeloma can be. One man had even booked his wife into the hotel but she could not make it. Another young man, and there were surprisingly quite a few, had a horror story to tell. He had been attending his doctor complaining of a bad back for some time and had been told not to play so much sport or to be careful with gardening, neither of which he did. Eventually when he was diagnosed, the myeloma had spread to his bones and he was wheelchair bound. It is a rare condition, there must be a lot of doctors who have never seen it. Just as perplexing is the cause of the illness. One possible clue is being investigated in America. A factory involved in tanning leather moved into a town and the incidence of myeloma shot up. There has to be a cause for this but, up till now, it has not been isolated. Once the researchers know the cause it may be easier to provide a cure.

The thing about July is that the football season is almost upon us. So where does that leave me? Despondent and bitter that my team were relegated on the last day of the season. Coventry were 9 to 1 to go down, and the bookies are never wrong, except in this case. Coventry did the usual thing when they are in trouble by starting their game 15/20 minutes after the other bottom teams, but they were allowed to get away with it. Be that as it may, we are down, and it is our fault. At one time we had nine first team players with long term injuries, and yet we did not replace them. An old banking maxim must surely apply. If your organisation is not doing well, be it a business, a scout troop, a football team, or whatever, there are three reasons. The first is the management, the second is the management, and the third is the management. I mean by that 'management' in the true sense, not just the team manager.

Things are going slowly, I think I am improving slowly, and I am confident that I will get no worse, but the non-myeloma problems are getting to me. I was talking to Paul, and I found it difficult to speak as if I were having a migraine attack. Over the years I have had migraine but never in this form. My brother did, and it looks as if my past problems may have altered my metabolism. In any event it only lasted for about 40 minutes but it was unusual, and I don't need anything else to worry about.

I tend to see the lunch time news broadcasts as I am at home quite often and it is surprising how many advances have been claimed for the treatment of all kinds of cancers but never my one. The problem is, nothing else is heard about them. One was very interesting and I can only describe it in the way it was reported. The procedure is to magnetise the myeloma cells, which meant that only the myeloma cells were hit by the chemo, enabling more to be used. Healthy tissues were left untouched, and the treatment seems to show a lot of promise. The patient had made a very quick and ostensibly full recovery, which is a ray of hope. Research is going on all over the world, but this one seems to warrant urgent attention.

My other pre-occupation is not proceeding very well. Sunderland started off badly, and have been trying to catch up all the time. We were being beaten by teams that our reserves should have taken care of. The underlying grouse is that we should not have been relegated and that makes it all the more bitter. The one thing to come out of it is that the new stadium is superb. There will never be another Roker Park for so many

Myeloma and me

of my boyhood memories are linked with it. We will just have to keep crawling up the league and hope that the top teams falter.

The year filters out and I am still keeping going, and was able to exchange letters with Helen Rollason. She has a worse cancer than mine and yet she is back reporting sport on the BBC. My attitude towards my myeloma has been to spit in its eye, she seems to have adopted Elton John's song 'I'm still standing' and with Gloria Gaynor's 'I will survive' there are a couple of cancer patients anthems all ready for Christmas. She is a gutsy lady, and I think it will be a very strong cancer to get her. I have also heard of a garden nurseryman in Scotland who is growing roses and for every one he sells he is giving a donation to leukaemia research, who are also researching into myeloma. I have bought one for all my family and it is called 'Ray of Hope'.

The big event in the latter stages of the year was our trip to Australia. My doctors had no objection, my insurance company had no objection, so off we went. I am aware of my neuralgia by now and how it affects me. This winter I have found that cold makes it worse and although I can usually sit without too much trouble, sliding from side to side causes mayhem. Aircraft seats are not the most comfortable, and I was expecting problems. As my TENS machine would be needed I decided that I had better show it to the cabin staff. I could see panic ensuing if someone saw me with my machine, with a battery, dials, wires and lights. I was amazed that they showed no interest, very strange. The flight was no problem, apart from showing Mr Bean every couple of hours and we enjoyed our stop over in Kuala Lumpur.

I love Australia but I am afraid that Sydney has caught the money bug. Everyone is trying to make money out of the Olympics and the city which I had really enjoyed just three years ago has lost its appeal. Andie and Steve are doing well and little Emily is amazing. When we were there, instead of a christening, a celebrant performed a naming ceremony. The celebrant is the equivalent of our registrars and the ceremony was performed in the back garden. Emily and the children from next door were about the only Australians there. Emily is a happy little girl, and has a habit of smiling at everyone she meets. One day we took her down to Sydney on the train and we sat opposite a real old grump and he was having to do with her. She worked on him; after about 10 minutes, he was forced to smile at her. If she is like this at one year old I wonder what another ten might bring. The Oz family Anderson are clearly loving the life over there and mentioned that we could probably sell our house in Sawbridgeworth and buy two over there, one for living, and the other for renting. The idea has great appeal especially as the temperature helped my pain. We shall see. I found out too late that the local hospital were having discussions on myeloma and it would have been interesting to hear their thoughts.

It all came to an end and we had to return to the cold of our winter and the proof that my neuralgia is badly affected by cold. Unfortunately there is nothing that can be realistically done for me. I have had the pills and had to stop because of the side effects, Ultra sound did not help, there is only my TENS machine which can dull the pain on a good day but never removes it. My only option, which I will never accept, is to open my spine and physically cut away the damaged nerve. That literally sends shivers down my spine, I can do without that and will struggle on as best I can. I saw Dr Marcus for my 6-monthly visit and he was pleased with how well I looked. After two weeks I had the results of the tests which were fine. I can look forward to the new year with reasonable confidence.

The first few weeks were spent on non medical matters, but which would have an effect on me. Our local court house was to be closed and although we fought a very good rearguard action, and I am sure won the argument, money prevailed, and the court was closed. It will have an effect on me as I can not always travel and now it would be a 35 mile round trip instead of six. The main point, though, is the defendants in cases, many of whom are on benefit, having to make a costly journey. This Government is pledged to maintain local justice; that principle has been destroyed once and for all.

I also did my pain threshold no good with my repeated trips up to the North East for home games. We have been gradually inching upwards and are within reach of the top. Just as last season, one game sticks out like a beacon. We needed to win one more game to be assured of promotion. I made sure that I could make it up to the North East, my family managed to get tickets and I was all set for a great day. Nottingham Forest were top, we were second, and Middlesbrough third, and admitting that they would probably have to settle for that. Our theme music as the team comes on to the pitch is 'Dance of the Knights', by Prokofiev, and whoever dreamed that up is a master. When the team arrives and the music plays the hairs on the back of the neck stand out. There is also a piece of music that is played when we score, 'I feel good', by James Brown, but in comparison it is so American and cheap, and it should be scrapped. The Sunderland fans are well able to show their pleasure when a goal is scored. This game was against Queen's Park Rangers, and we were excellent. The football I love, with orthodox wingers playing well, crosses swinging over, it was a pleasure to be there. With eight minutes to go, and cruising along at 2-0, our defence went to sleep, and we drew 2-2. This meant that we missed automatic promotion and landed up in the accursed play-offs.

For those not fully conversant with the system it is an abomination. Three teams are promoted, the top two go up automatically, and the next four play off for the third spot. This can mean and has meant that the team finishing 6th and 20 points behind the leader, can go up. It is an absolute disgrace and I fail to see why professional players do not refuse to take part in them. Just because someone has the chance to make a lot of money and the FA is too gutless to stop it teams have to go through this tawdry spectacle every year. In the event, our game was probably the best seen at Wembley for many years, but that is not the point. Scrap the squalid play offs, what a slogan. This left us still in Division One and who knows what effect this will have on the players next season. We shall have to see.

The year drifts on and apart from 'Miracle' cancer cures reported on the TV and in the press nothing seems to happen. This is clearly because of the time delay between a possible idea and the drug being perfected. My own problems are really concerned with my neuralgia which is very difficult to predict. The pain is there all the time and as the damaged nerve band starts at the breast bone and carries round under my arms to the middle of my spine it is very difficult to sit, or sleep. My TENS machine dulls the pain down but, if I use it every day, I get used to it and then have to stop for a while which is annoying. The main thing which sent me off to the Doctor's was another episode like I had last year. It is strange, with speech and vision being affected, but the whole episode lasting about 50 minutes. I had three of these attacks within three weeks and ended up going to see Dr Wilkinson which is fine, as he is a nice man, but here we go on another mystery tour. The symptoms are very similar to a stroke but the very short duration of the attacks tend to belie this.

I had to attend Addenbrooke's, as nothing was apparent from the original consultation and apart from the chaotic scenes on the ward due to a shortage of staff it went well. In my experience of the NHS the treatments are fine but they are so busy they miss out the niceties, like knowing who you are. It would be nice if they would tell the patient how long they would have to wait, where the toilets are, simple things like that. In my case, I had to have five different tests in different parts of the building, and we were left to wonder what was happening next most of the time. There were various checks of veins, arteries, heart valves, and possible clots, and the 'piece de resistance' the MR scan. This was used to test my brain and is a little claustrophobic and noisy but we were on our way home again by 6 o'clock, a nine hour day. The test would have to be pored over and analysed but the instant result tests showed that I had no problems with my heart or arteries, no blood clots, which left the odds lengthening on my brain. Still, there is nothing to do but wait, which is something I am not good at. My appointments with Dr Marcus are no problem but the waiting for two weeks for the results make me jumpy even though I am certain that everything is going well.

At least there was no reason to delay our holiday, I now had two consultants, my G.P. and my insurance company to consider, but I had no problems from any of them. We were on holiday during the World Cup and it was odd watching football from our balcony in the Costa Brava with the various nationalities groaning or cheering as the games were played. The World Cup is not my favourite tournament as it is so much over-hyped but the football was not too bad. I think part of it was that I was having my usual apprehension over my neurological results. The weather was glorious and I noticed after four days that my neuralgia pain was easing which is something I had noticed before. If heat is what is required, roll on the sun, which is not bad, as before coming away we booked up for Corfu at the back of September.

On our return from holiday the report from Dr Marcus was waiting and things as I suspected, are doing fine with another consultation to be arranged in December. We had an agonising wait for Dr Wilkinson, my neurologist, but we eventually went to see him. He sees patients at home and it is one of those chocolate box thatched houses and looks delightful. His report, however, was that after checking every part of me that could cause the problem he had found nothing. I must admit that I always hope for something very minor which can be corrected easily but no such luck. The very good thing is that my brain, heart, lungs, veins and arteries have been meticulously tested, and are fine. Not fine for a 59 year old man after having chemo, but fine. Dr Wilkinson is pleased of course, but suggests that I keep an eye on my cholesterol, which is fine at the moment and take an aspirin every day which will make sure the blood stays fluid and that is that. Out of yet another lions den. Now I know how Houdini felt.

The year carries on, I have by now forgotten my scare over my neurological episode and I have had no further problems, and we come to August, which can only mean one thing, the start of the football season. I have often been asked how it came about that I am such an ardent supporter of Sunderland, and it is just Sunderland. In my view, football as I knew it as a boy has gone, greed, dishonesty and hype have taken over, but Sunderland is totally different With me it started when I was nine and I felt right from then that I belonged. The whole town was engrossed in the game and a lot of people could remember just before the war when we were one of the giants of the game. It certainly affected my schooling. My mother was called up to the school once as they were concerned that on occasions they could do nothing with me. It took my mother a while to realise that it was when we lost at home the previous Saturday.

If a boy grows up in this atmosphere it is inevitable that he becomes a fan. For true devotion, I maintain that also you must have played the game, even at a poor level, as I did. My friends are surprised that I can not stand rugby and I think the answer is that I have never played it and know nothing about it. I can never fathom how anyone can support a club over which they have no affinity. David Mellor changed from supporting Fulham to Chelsea, and for the life of me I can not understand how anyone can do that. It is like having a divorce, but then luckily I know nothing about that either. I know that shortly after we were engaged June asked my mother how I came to be so devoted to the team. My mother replied with an astute comment that if I showed such love for a football team, just think what I will feel for my family. I grew up with the moods of the town being linked to the performance of the team. Many years later, when we beat Leeds in the 1973 Cup Final, the factories who were on piece work noticed a sharp rise in production. I repeat, if all of this is missing, I can not see how a true devotion can be found. One of the Sunderland fan magazines is called 'A Love Supreme' and that says it all. Having said all of that there is no doubt that if I had been born 12 miles further north I would have been an avid Newcastle fan. I can't quite believe I have written that, but it is true. Apart from the odd 100 or so mental cases, the Sunderland fans are just the same as the Newcastle fans and I have the same feeling. I can not believe that someone from Torquay or Wales can adopt Manchester United and be as fervent as me, I just don't think it is possible. You must have lived it, suffered the bad times, played it, and loved it.

I have seen a couple of the early games and although we have lots of injuries we are playing well with no apparent hangover from the nonsense of the play off final. In my contempt for this parody of football justice, I have even written to Bob Murray, the Sunderland Chairman, to see if he can do anything to get it scrapped. I would suspect that he can do nothing, where money is to be found, fairness and sportsmanship go out of the window. Even if I had wanted to, I could never get away from it. We went on holiday to Corfu and the courier supported Atletico Madrid and he says they play in the famous Red and White. I even have red and white blood corpuscles.

To more important matters. We went to the myeloma seminar at Southampton amid appalling weather. Someone has got this wrong. Our last one was in Edinburgh and the weather was glorious, now we come down to the deep south and it was truly awful. It started off sadly. The man who could not bring his wife to Edinburgh reported that she had just died, and he delivered a eulogy which left no eye dry or any throat without constriction. As at Edinburgh, the specialists said again that there was still no cure and that mortality rates had not improved. One went a step further and said that because of bone damage, the average myeloma patient ends up two inches smaller, thank you for that, it was really appreciated.

Into this scenario, we needed hope. Up stepped Professor Freda Stevenson and she was like a shaft of light. First of all she had a beautiful speaking voice, and her descriptions of her work of gene therapy was absorbing, and gave hope to all. Her work involves using the DNA to isolate the gene which governs the immune system and, in effect, switches it on to attack the invading cells. The way she described it as a simple, cheap procedure, gave me visions of doing it on the kitchen work top at 50 pence a time. She did say that her procedure works on mice, how come mice get protection from diseases before we do? The procedure is applicable to many forms of cancer, not just myeloma, and it sounds really exciting.. She gave me more hope that any other speaker at one of these functions and I am grateful for it. If I were a betting man I would be looking for the odds for Prof. Stevenson to beat myeloma and be awarded the Nobel Peace Prize.

I have mentioned fairness once or twice but here is another example. Back to football again. We are playing well, and we lost for the first time on November 21st, which was the 25th game. The comment from the BBC, precisely nothing. They are supposed to be the British Broadcasting Corporation not an apologist for the Premier League or a public relations firm for the London teams. This is what will help kill football. The non Premier teams get so little attention that they will lose heart as well as money. I remember when, after every news broadcast, the results of the games played that evening are read out. Now it is just the Premier League, and it is disgraceful. Have not Rotherham, Stockport or Carlisle fans a right to hear how their team is doing? Anyway, the year is drifting on and the weather is getting worse as is my damned neuralgia.

I am almost at peace with my TENS machine. I work from home two days a week, which I prefer. I still have my family and friends and a wonderful little grand-daughter with her own Australian passport in which it is marked that she is not allowed to work in Britain. We are planning our next trip to Australia so that is something else to look forward to. I still sit as a magistrate and carry on with my school governorship, so on the surface, very little has changed if you forget the intervening three years. My myeloma appears to be beaten as the readings are entirely stable and as long as this is the case, I can look forward to many years of remission by which time someone will have found a lasting cure. Research is being carried out all over the world and it could come at any time, but I would love it to come from Freda Stevenson.

I now have the pain from the post herpetic neuralgia, my eyes are prone to soreness. I put this down to the time when my tear ducts were not working. Now if I am in a car with the air fan blasting at my eyes I get sore eyes for days. Although I can hear well, some days I find it difficult to separate one noise from many. This may be nerve damage, we will have to see. My doctor noticed an odd thing the other day. After my period of not eating the ligaments and muscles in my jaw have wasted, and I can not open my mouth very wide, and there is a flat section near both ears. My voice gets weak after a while, and very husky, which I put down to the period when my vocal cords were damaged. I find now that I can't sing. I couldn't before because of lack of ability, now it seems to be a weakness. Apart from the above, my stamina is suspect, intense concentration tires me out, and I have the vague feeling that I am not the lad I used to be. I think that the chemo wreaked havoc on my system and a few of my faculties have received permanent damage. As they say, chemo saves your life, but it murders you. This is the sum total of what ails me now, and when I compare the time when I tipped the scales at 7st 5, had not eaten for nine months and had not spoken above a whisper for six, I am well satisfied. I have been down into the depths, and have withstood all that myeloma can throw at me and I have come through it all. Life is good.

EPILOGUE

Over the course of this book, the fortunes of Sunderland AFC have varied widely. From the euphoria of promotion to the Premier League with an amazing 105 points and 91 goals we are still there. Over the last two seasons we have declined, Peter Reid has gone, and nails are starting to be bitten. Relegation was a close run thing last season, but my view of the Premier League has not altered. I regard it as being exploitative, greedy, over-hyped and contemptuous of lower clubs. It will only get worse.

I have been forced to realise that my Post Herpatic Neuralgia has become worse, particularly in damp, cold weather. Whilst I continue to use my TENS machine, its ability to reduce the pain has lessened. At various times I have tried other treatments, but they have been no help. I have now accepted that the condition is permanent and that the unpleasant effects it has on my life will remain.

On the myeloma front, things are going well. I now have annual checkups, and Dr Marcus is pleased with my progress. It tool over a year for my illness to be described as being in remission. Now, my reports have included comments like: Virtual Complete Remission", and "Excellent Remission". I will settle for that.

Neither a cause or a cure has been found, but I am convinced that a cure will one day be perfected. Scientists are working steadily to find a cure, and I am sure that they will succeed as more research is undertaken, and the frontiers of knowledge pushed out. I hope that it is soon.

Ray Grummett
October 2002